Alternative Therapies

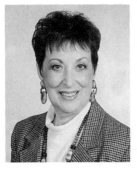

Rena J. Gordon, PhD, is Research Lecturer in family and community medicine at the University of Arizona College of Medicine and Adjunct Professor of geography at Arizona State University. Committed to improving health care services for special populations, her research has assisted the delivery of health care in rural communities in Arizona. She authored the *Arizona Rural Health Provider Atlas* (1984, 1987), which has been selected by the U.S. Department of State for distribution to overseas organizations involved in epidemiological studies, and has served as a model for Florida's health care atlas. Her research on intraurban physician location, malpractice and rural obstetric service, maternal and child health, long-term care and elder services, primary care services in underserved areas, and health services delivery in Cuba has appeared in journals and as book chapters. She is Contributing Editor to the *Encyclopedia of Complementary Health Practices.* Dr. Gordon also has published on health policy issues and on the health services delivery system and healing practices in Cuba.

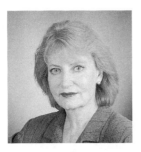

Barbara Cable Nienstedt, DPA, is Director of The Research Network, a consulting firm specializing in research design and evaluation. As a research methodologist, Dr. Nienstedt has been responsible for the reliability, validity, and analysis of numerous large-scale projects in diverse government agencies, working extensively with federal and state courts. Her research experience in the political and legal aspects of alternative health have included evaluations of regulatory agencies and boards, demographic and lifestyle influences on health, cancer clusters, and cross-cultural aspects of alternative health, including conducting interviews at a major teaching hospital in traditional Chinese medicine in Guilin, China. Currently, Dr. Nienstedt is working as research consultant to an organization of medical doctors interested in testing an experimental device. She has also been appointed to the Professional Advisory Board of the largest provider of home health care in North America.

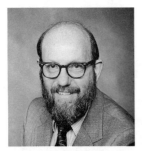

Wilbert M. Gesler, PhD, is George J. Kane Professor of Geography at the University of North Carolina, Chapel Hill. His main research interest is in the geography of health. Current work includes the investigation of therapeutic landscapes or places that have achieved a lasting reputation for healing, the role of language in health encounters in places, and the cultural geography of health behavior in a rural town in North Carolina. In addition to conducting research in the United States, Europe, and Africa, he has also published a book on the cultural geography of health care and has edited books on the geography of health in North America, geographic methods for investigating health issues along the rural-urban continuum, and putting health into place.

Alternative Therapies

Expanding Options in Health Care

Rena J. Gordon, PhD

Barbara Cable Nienstedt, DPA

Wilbert M. Gesler, PhD

Springer Publishing Company

Springer Publishing Company, Inc.
536 Broadway
New York, NY 10012-3955

Cover design by Margaret Dunin
Acquisitions Editor: Bill Tucker
Production Editor: Kathleen Kelly

98 99 00 01 02 / 5 4 3 2 1

Library of Congress Cataloging-in-Publication-Data

Alternative therapies : exploring options in health care / [edited by]
    Rena J. Gordon, Barbara Cable Nienstedt, Wilbert M. Gesler.
        p.   cm.
    Includes bibliographical references and index.
    ISBN 0-8261-1164-5
    1. Alternative medicine.   2. Medical care—Utilization.
I. Gordon, Rena J.   II. Nienstedt, Barbara Cable.   III. Gesler,
Wilbert M., 1941–
    [DNLM: 1. Alternative Medicine—trends.   WB 890 A4662 1998]
    R733.A516   1998
    615.5—dc21
    DNLM/DLC
    for Library of Congress   97-41351
                                                                      CIP

Printed in the United States of America

*The publisher does not advocate the use of any particular remedy contained in
this book and is not responsible for any adverse effects or consequences resulting from the use of any of the procedures or remedies presented in this book.*

Contents

Contributors

Leonard D. Baer, MS, is pursuing a PhD degree in geography at the University of North Carolina and works as a research assistant at the Cecil G. Sheps Center for Health Services Research. His current research focuses on whether international medical graduates fill gaps for physician shortages by practicing in rural, underserved areas. A medical geographer with a master's degree from Virginia Tech, his thesis was awarded the Jacques M. May prize of the Medical Geography Specialty Group, Association of American Geographers. He has worked in the past as a health policy analyst for the state of Maryland and as a consultant in survey research.

Barbara Stevens Barnum, RN, PhD, FAAN, is Professor at the Columbia University School of Nursing and Editor of *Nursing Leadership Forum.* A Certified *Reiki* practitioner, Dr. Barnum has recently written *Spirituality in Nursing: From Traditional to New Age.* This book joins others she has written on nursing theory and administration and on writing and getting published. Dr. Barnum is a Fellow of the American Academy of Nursing and has done extensive national and international consultation in nursing and health care administration, including an 8-year term as consultant to the U.S. Air Force Surgeon General.

Kristen S. Borré, PhD, MPH, is an Assistant Clinical Professor and Director of Community Health Studies in the Department of Family Medicine and Adjunct Assistant Professor of anthropology, East Carolina University. With an MPH in nutrition and a PhD in anthropology, she has studied cultural models of health and diet among Canadian Inuit, plant use among the eastern Arctic Inuit, and ecological models of diet. Her current research includes public health assessment in eastern North Carolina; the attitudes, perceptions, and beliefs of local health providers concerning telemedicine; concepts and practices of mental health care among rural primary care physicians; and occupational and environmental risks to health among North Carolina crabbers and their families.

Jerry Calkins, PhD, MD, is a Professor of clinical anesthesiology at the University of Arizona, and Adjunct Professor of engineering in the Department of Chemical, Bio and Materials Engineering at Arizona State University, and Chairman of the Department of Anesthesiology at Maricopa Medical Center. He is active in the application of technology to anesthesia and is particularly interested in new modalities of treatment for patients with chronic pain. He has completed the course on acupuncture for physicians at UCLA and has chaired several national conferences, including the recent meeting on acupuncture sponsored by the NIH Office of Alternative Medicine and the Food and Drug Administration. His current research interests are the mechanisms of acupuncture and its application to surgical anesthesia.

Ronald L. Caplan, PhD, is an Assistant Professor of public health at Richard Stockton College of New Jersey. A health economist by training, he specializes in health policy and planning and recently co-authored a book on health care reform. Dr. Caplan also specializes in the economics of alternative health care. Over the past 20 years he has published and lectured widely on this topic, focusing especially on chiropractic. He was an economic advisor to the American Chiropractic Association in the 1980s. Currently, Dr. Caplan teaches a seminar on alternative health care at Richard Stockton College.

Charles M. Good, Jr. PhD, is Professor of geography at Virginia Tech, in Blacksburg, Virginia. He teaches courses in medical geography, African development, and world regions. Dr. Good has conducted field research on traditional medical and healing systems in Kenya, including linkages with biomedicine. He has ongoing interests in ethnomedicine and medical cultures, community-based health care, the ecology of health, the HIV/AIDs around the world. Currently, he is preparing a book about the African missionary frontier in colonial Malawi. This study examines how the introduction of lake steamers and European medicine by the Universities' Mission to central Africa influenced spatial relations, health care, and society on and near Lake Malawi.

Mary M. Hale, DPA, is Assistant Professor in the Division of Social and Policy Sciences at the University of Texas at San Antonio. She teaches courses in public policy and health care in the public administration and political science programs. Prior to university service, Dr. Hale had a 13-year career in behavioral health care and administration. Her research interests include civic participation in policy-making, work analysis of recruitment and retention of health care professionals in rural areas, and long-term care utilization. She is published in the fields of public administration and women in politics and is currently involved in researching alternative methods for prioritizing funding of health and human services. Dr. Hale is co-editor of *Gender, Bureaucracy, and Democracy: Careers and Equal Opportunity in the Public Sector* and is a contributing author to numerous articles and books.

Jill M. Hyatt, BA, is currently completing a master's degree in public administration at the University of Texas at San Antonio and plans to pursue doctoral studies in this area. She is a former Equal Employment Opportunity and fair housing investigator and is interested in researching these areas further in her graduate studies. Her other research interests include health and human services and immigration policies.

Clarissa T. Kimber, PhD, is Professor of geography at Texas A&M University in College Station, Texas. Long interested in the use of plants as medicine, she also studies folk medical systems and their integration with biomedical systems in various countries. Her interest in plant–people relationships in the tropics led to a book on the changing plant geographies in Martinique. Dr. Kimber was a Fulbright scholar at National Taiwan University in 1996, where she collaborated on a study at the use and sale of herbal preparations in Taipei, Taiwan.

Evan W. Kligman, MD, is Professor and Head of the Department of Family Medicine at the University of Iowa College of Medicine. His degrees include a BA in anthropology from UCLA and an MD from the University of Arizona, where he completed a family practice residency program, general preventive medicine residency practicum year, and faculty development fellowship. Kligman was a 1993 U.S. Public Health Service Primary Care Policy Fellow. He participated in developing the Program in Integrative Medicine at the University of Arizona and is coordinator for integrative medicine curriculum in the Department of Family medicine at the University of Iowa. He has served as co-chair of the Society of Teachers of Family Medicine work group on health promotion and disease prevention.

Joan D. Koss-Chioino, PhD, is a medical anthropologist who works in the fields of anthropology, psychiatry, and psychology. Her primary interest is the treatment of illness and emotional problems, especially in Hispanic cultures. She is Professor of anthropology at Arizona State University and Adjunct Professor of psychiatry and neurology at Tulane Medical Center in New Orleans. Currently, she is conducting treatment research with Mexican American youth and families in Arizona. Her publications include studies of women as both healers and patients in Puerto Rico and psychotherapeutic interventions with ethnic minority children and adolescents.

Alan Rice Osborn is a PhD, is a recent recipient of a doctorate in geography from the University of Oregon. His research has focused on the spatial and distributional aspects of health and health care. His research interests include alternative medicine, biogeography, geostatistics, and the geographical analysis of literature. He received the Jacques M. May prize of the Medical Geography Specialty Group, Association of American Geographers, for his master's thesis on the distribution of alternative health care practitioners in San Diego, California.

Dona Schneider, PhD, MPH, is Associate Professor in Rutgers University's Department of Urban Studies and Community Health. As a medical geographer and epidemiologist, Dr. Schneider's research interests and expertise include the study of mortality, morbidity, and high-risk behaviors, especially for children, minorities, and selected high-risk groups. Recent works include two books, *American Childhood: Risks and Realities* and *Environmentally Devastated Neighborhoods: Perceptions, Policies, and Realities,* co-authored with Dr. Michael Greenberg. Dr. Schneider has also recently published a book chapter on childhood cancer risks for the Pennsylvania Academy of Science, as well as multiple articles on health and policy issues.

Gail Silverstein, DPA, is Vice President, of Health Plans, Maricopa Integrated Health Systems, in Phoenix, Arizona. She is an adjunct professor in the School of Health Administration and Policy at Arizona State University and also has taught public sector marketing of health care at Arizona State and Florida International University in Miami. Previous research has included studies in the area of physician satisfaction and participation in managed care and Medicaid programs. She received a Doctor of Public Administration degree from Arizona State University.

James L. Wilson, PhD, is a medical geographer with academic interests in historical epidemiology, infectious diseases, and demography. He has studied 18th- and 19th-century smallpox epidemics and medicine in Finland. Currently, he is a research associate at East Carolina University's Center for Health Services Research and Development, where he works on issues concerning medically underserved areas in eastern North Carolina. He holds a PhD degree from the University of North Carolina, Chapel Hill, and is also an Adjunct Professor of Geography at Eastern Carolina University.

Foreword

Alternative Therapies: Expanding Options in Health Care, is not a typical book on alternative medicine because it is not written by diehard advocates of alternative medicine. Rather, it is authored by keen observers of an emerging health movement—it is written primarily by nonclinicians. Although there is one chapter written by a physician and another by a nurse, the majority of this work is authored by specialists from a wide diversity of academic disciplines, including geography, anthropology, engineering, health economics, public policy, public administration, epidemiology, and marketing.

The representation from the various academic disciplines gives the book a multi-layer view of the alternative medicine movement. Most books on the subject describe the history, present status, principles, research, and clinical applications of specific treatment modalities. This book does this and more. It also provides the cultural, social, demographic, political, economic, and legal implications of alternative therapies. It describes the emerging difficulties that present licensing and other regulatory measures created for this new movement, and it describes various federal and state efforts to change laws so that this movement can continue to grow in a way that still provides consumer protection.

Many of the practices termed "alternative" in the United States are part of established medical systems in other parts of the world. For example, it would be incorrect to refer to acupuncture as "alternative medicine" in China when you consider that most of that country's population uses it as a primary form of health care. It would likewise seem strange to refer to homeopathic medicine as "alternative medicine" in Europe when almost 40% of French doctors and 20% of German doctors use these natural medicines in their practice, when 42% of British physicians refer patients to homeopathic doctors, and 45% of Dutch physicians consider homeopathic medicines to be effective. Even the World Health Organization estimates that 80% of the world's population uses "traditional medicine" as their primary health care ("traditional medicine" is defined as indigenous folk medicines—this ultimately comprises much of what is today called "alternative medicine").

The above statistics may question the appropriateness of the term "alternative medicine"; however, what is also true is that what is called "conventional medicine" in the United States and other industrialized countries today is the dominant medical treatment that pervades contemporary care given by medical doctors. In this sense, the treatments and approaches to health that are described in this book are certainly "alternative."

When one considers learning about the subject of alternative medicine, it is important to know that this field does not simply represent medicines and modalities of treatment different from those used in conventional medical care. The field of alternative medicine also represents a different paradigm to understanding health and disease. For instance, it is common for alternative practitioners to recognize that a person does not simply have a disease that is localized in the heart, liver, kidney, or any other specific part of the body, but that person's disease is a part of a body-mind pattern or syndrome of illness.

Inherent in this different approach is also the recognition of the importance to providing individualized treatment to a person and her or his unique pattern of illness. In alternative medicine there is a respect for the wisdom of the body-mind. Instead of assuming that symptoms of illness are "wrong," which then need to be treated, controlled, managed, or suppressed as is commonly the goal in conventional biomedicine, users of the various alternatives therapies attempt to nourish and nurture the wisdom of the body-mind so that it can heal itself.

The most famous words that Hippocrates, the father of medicine, ever said were, "First, do no harm." Sadly, however, physicians who specialize in conventional biomedicine have not yet fully understood what Hippocrates meant by the word, "First." When they do, they will seek out and use many of the "alternative" therapies discussed in this book. When this happens, which probably will be in the near future, it will no longer be necessary to call it "alternative" medicine.

Dana Ullman, MPH
Founder and Director
Homeopathic Educational Services
Berkeley, California

Acknowledgments

My greatest gratitude goes to Leonard Gordon for his critical editorial comments, creative suggestions, patience, and unwavering support. I would like to thank Mary McPherson for her valued computer assistance throughout the final stages of manuscript preparation; Katherine Matas, who led me to see the need to add a nursing chapter; Augusto Ortiz, whose teaching and holistic practice of medicine planted a seed for the development of this book; David P. Williams III for his writing suggestions; Shirley Ogle for sharing research materials on business aspects of alternative therapies; Christa Hughes and Joanne P. Stein for copyediting; and Bill Tucker of Springer Publishing Company for guiding the book through to production. The love and encouragement of my family and friends and their keen interest in the topic helped keep me on track to complete this long project.

R.J.G.

I wish to acknowledge Peter B. Chowka and Michael S. Evers, JD, for sharing their expertise and experience with me, despite more critical demands on their time.

B.C.N.

The authors of chapter 9 would like to thank Nydia I. Guerrero for her help in reviewing the literature on alternative health practices among Mexican Americans. Ms. Guerrero is an MPA student and research assistant at the University of Texas at San Antonio.

J.M.H. and M.M.H.

List of Tables

List of Figures

PART I
Introduction

Our dilemma is that we hate change and love it at the same time;
what we want is for things to remain the same but get better.
—Sidney Harris

Part One surveys the history of American medicine and suggests reasons for the recent trend by an increasing number of people to use alternative therapies. It also recommends a model to bring order and better understanding of the diversity in approach among the bewildering array of alternative therapies. This section provides a basic background for the remainder of the book.

In chapter 1, Wil Gesler and Rena Gordon propose reasons that people are going beyond biomedicine to treat some health care problems. Reasons that alternative therapies are attracting attention include the high cost of biomedicine, the emphasis on cure of disease rather than on lifestyle change and prevention, the focus on high technology and toxic drugs that could have harmful side effects, the dismissal of the role of spirituality and humanity in healing, and the limitations in dealing with chronic health problems of an aging American population. The role of aging baby boomers in creating demand for alternative therapies is discussed. To understand the present trend better, historical background to 19th-century medical pluralism, which was superseded in the 20th-century by the singular dominance of biomedicine, is presented. The large number of people using alternative therapies suggests a return to medical pluralism in the 21st century.

In chapter 2, Barbara Cable Nienstedt tackles the essential task of describing what alternative medicine is and mentions individuals and groups in this diverse category. She explains the use of the term *alternative*, and defines it for the purpose of this book; she also defines both complementary and holistic medicine. The core of this chapter is a four-part model of complementary medicine that categorizes several dozen specific practices under the headings of either biomedicine or one of three types of alternative medicine: body healing, mind/spirit, and cross-cultural. The point is made that some alternative therapies are here to stay, others are likely to fade into obscurity, and still others may return after a period of dormancy. Also, it is noted that alternative therapies represent very complex systems of beliefs and practices and therefore are best understood only after long periods of study.

1

Alternative Therapies: Why Now?

Wilbert M. Gesler and Rena J. Gordon

> It is better to know some of the questions
> than all of the answers.
> —James Thurber

A new option in health care is exploding on the American scene. A significant reality in American society today is the increasing use of therapies that are not part of Western biomedicine. Most readers of this book either will have tried an alternative remedy or will know someone who has. The *New England Journal of Medicine* (Eisenberg et al., 1993) reported that fully one third of the adult American population used an alternative therapy and one third of these went to an alternative practitioner for treatment. The question is, why is there such a dramatic change in mind-set?

A major reason for the new mind-set is dissatisfaction with elements of Western biomedicine, the dominant medical paradigm, that focuses on disease and its cure by surgery, pharmaceutical remedies, and sophisticated technology. The list of complaints is lengthy. Although biomedicine has been quite effective in dealing with infectious and contagious diseases, it is often ineffective in curing chronic problems, such as heart disease, the major cause of illness and death in the United States. Also, the focus of biomedicine is on cure rather than prevention, whereas many people believe that emphasis on prevention would be far more cost-effective in the long run. In addition, many biomedical cures are questioned because they have been found to have serious side effects. In fact, biomedicine has often been accused of being iatrogenic; that is, health problems are induced inadvertently by a physician or a treatment.

For many people, biomedicine has a stuffy, austere, cold, and uncaring image. Physicians and other medical practitioners, it is thought, treat patients with sterilized gloves and keep them at a distance; they do not treat people as human beings with feelings (Hulke, 1979). As biomedicine continues to emphasize high-tech innovation, the cost of care escalates, often beyond the ability of many Americans to pay. Indeed, the cost of medical care has increased faster than inflation for many years. Meanwhile, we are currently witnessing cutbacks in government spending for health care. Another problem is the maldistribution of the benefits of biomedicine. Many, such as the working poor who do not qualify for Medicaid benefits and yet cannot afford health insurance, are left without even basic care, let alone care using high-tech treatment.

The second major reason for the new mind-set can be traced to the aging of the baby boom generation. Baby boomers, those born between 1946 and 1964, are now beginning to turn 50. Cheryl Russell, in her book *The Master Trend: How the Baby Boom Generation Is Remaking America* (1993), claims that much of the upheaval in America today (including problems stemming from divorce, drug abuse, materialism, a lack of duty and commitment, and an unwillingness to sacrifice) is due to the attitudes and values of baby boomers, who now dominate the demographic landscape. The existence, thinking, and behavior of baby boomers have had and will continue to have important health care implications. The first batch of the 77 million baby boomers is beginning to hit the half-century mark. As the dominant baby boom cohort ages, it faces a myriad of health problems and will require more health care. Already obsessed with their own bodies, this population is waging a battle against the aging process itself. Baby boomers are on a constant search for whatever will turn back the hands of time. This helps to explain why the trend toward using alternative therapies is occurring now.

A third major reason for the new mind-set surfaces as we witness a genuine desire for wellness, which many are attempting to satisfy outside biomedicine (Kearney & Rosch, 1985). Many people clearly respond to the positive aspects of alternative health care. A major difference one finds in comparing biomedical and alternative treatments is the amount of time alternative practitioners spend with their patients and the emphasis they put on healer-patient interactions (Hinton, 1983). Others seek out the spiritual element in alternative healing, which they find missing in biomedicine. Although healing and religion usually were tightly integrated throughout most of history, modern medicine tends to separate them. Others who have turned to alternative therapies prefer the emphasis on prevention rather than cure, point to successes in many cases, and enjoy the relative ease of access. People are *pragmatic*. They vote with their feet, and they are voting more and more for alternatives.

The nature of health care in America is changing. People are taking more responsibility for their own health. Significant numbers of people are using alternative therapies, and significant amounts of money are being spent in this arena. Alternative medicine is becoming a competitive player in the health care marketplace. When there are competing medical systems, the phenomenon is called *medical pluralism.* It means that, in most times and places, people have a choice about what kind of practitioners they will use. Pluralism arises from the contact between different cultures, social change, and competing ideas about what disease is and what appropriate treatments should be (e.g., biomedicine and Chinese medicine are both prevalent in China today).

Many people use more than one medical system, depending on their particular problem, current beliefs, and advice from others; that is, people look for what they think will help them most in any specific situation. Someone suffering from acute low back pain, for example, can seek drug treatments and surgery from the biomedical system, adjustments from a chiropractor, relief from pain from an acupuncturist, massage therapy, and numerous other remedies. We should not be surprised by this "shopping around" behavior. Many people search for the best bargain or the item that best suits their fancy when they look for goods and services. Shopping for health care carries with it a different imperative, however, because it is the most important service in maintaining one's health. It differs from shopping for material goods and services in another way, because when one needs health care, one is not always in the position to shop—one could be very ill and need emergency care. Furthermore, health is a fragile, complex, and little understood commodity. The remedy that works for one person often does not work for another. In our individualistic society, people look for what is right for them, and they critically examine what is available.

Having knowledge is necessary to examine available options critically. This book provides a framework into which information can be sorted for examination. We recognize that no one piece of research or book can bring order out of all the information available on alternative practices. However, we can ask some basic questions. How can we make sense out of a bewildering array of alternative therapies? What factors have contributed to the increase in use in recent years? What role do federal and state policies play in advancing or restricting access to alternatives? How is demand for natural products and alternative therapies operationalized in the medical marketplace? Are alternative providers concentrated geographically? What role does health insurance coverage play in advancing access to alternative therapies? What differences do culture and ethnicity make in choices of alternative therapies? What are the policy implications for biomedical personnel? What changes are occurring in medical schools and in nursing schools? How are health policymakers responding to the expanding options? The purpose of this book is to address these questions.

The movement toward alternatives deserves both a respectful hearing and a critical analysis (Alster, 1989). We must debate the relative strengths and weaknesses of biomedicine and alternative medicine, search for what works and what does not, determine what increases or decreases costs, and discover what is quackery and what is genuine. At the same time, we should heed the warning that Wardwell (1963) gave: "We can reach no final judgment concerning relationships between the various health professions, because social pressures toward change continually arise both within and outside these professions" (p. 214). For example, observe how doctors of osteopathy (DOs), once shunned by the biomedical profession, have negotiated their way into the biomedical fold.

In the remainder of this chapter a background to the current health care situation will be presented as it relates to alternative medicine. First, a history of the competition between biomedicine and alternative medicine in the 19th and 20th centuries is summarized briefly to clarify more fully their relative position today. Second, the magnitude of the shift toward alternative care is documented. The chapter concludes with an outline of the organization of the rest of the book.

HOW DID THE MEDICAL SYSTEMS
IN AMERICA GET THIS WAY?

An understanding of the present health care situation and also of what the future might hold must entail a look at what has happened in the past (Kleinman, 1980). Looking at what has gone before helps us to recognize that health care practices are contingent on historical circumstances, such as what diseases were prevalent, what cultural practices were common, and what economic conditions were present. It helps us to realize that much of what is touted as "new" in alternative medicine is not really new at all but has been practiced for centuries. A historical viewpoint also makes us consider how and why health care practices have changed.

Although the many forms of medicine that have been practiced in America can be traced back to the time of Hippocrates, this discussion begins with the 19th century, when a host of therapies were vying for the attention of consumers. During most of the 19th century, biomedicine did not hold the dominant status it enjoys today; in fact, physicians held a fairly low status in the eyes of most people.

Although some Americans used biomedical doctors in the 19th century, many people were just as likely to patronize a diverse group of healers. People often avoided the drastic measures (such as bleeding, drugs that induced vomiting and purges, and irritants that blistered the skin) that doctors were promoting in the Age of Heroic Medicine (around 1780–1850) and were attracted to the claims made by alternative healers that their cures were natural (Alster, 1989). Quacks of all types abounded in both biomedicine and alternative medicine. There was also substantial competition from health crusades, religious healing, and folk medicine. At the same time, practitioners of homeopathy, chiropractic, and other alternatives were struggling to achieve professional status. (For an overview of this colorful history, see *Other Healers: Unorthodox Medicine in America* [Gevitz, 1988]).

It is generally agreed that germ theory, or the discovery that certain organisms caused specific diseases, was an early factor operating in favor of biomedicine toward the end of the 19th century (Wallis & Morley, 1976). Biomedical practitioners seized the opportunity to claim that theirs was the only medical practice based on truly scientific principles. They reviled and ridiculed their medical opponents as quacks and charlatans. Now, coming into the 20th century, they were able to legitimize themselves and marginalize alternative healers (Gevitz, 1988). Examples of this legitimation of biomedicine at the expense of alternative healers follow. The Pure Food and Drug Act of 1906 set standards of purity for food and drugs to help prohibit manufacturers from adulterating or misbranding their products. It was the Sherley Amendments of 1912 that made unlawful any false statement on the labels of foods and drugs (Burrow, 1963). These amendments helped to eliminate remedies and drugs falsely claiming therapeutic effects. The American Medical Association stopped carrying advertisements for these medicines in its journal and worked to enhance the professional status of its members. Abraham Flexner (1910), a man outside the medical profession and brother of the head of the Rockefeller Institute, reported on the state of all medical schools, which led to the establishment of biomedical standards for education in those schools and also licensing boards. It became difficult, if not impossible, for nonbiomedical practitioners to obtain licenses. Biomedicine was becoming the dominant medical system.

Alternative practitioners did not give ground easily, however. The criticisms biomedicine leveled at them were answered in kind. Alternative healers often called biomedical practitioners quacks and accused them of making people dependent on drugs (Gevitz, 1988). Furthermore, they claimed that they too used scientific practices and were often successful in curing diseases, particularly chronic problems. Unorthodox practitioners claimed that the biomedical professions created a monopoly and that their restrictive licensing laws deprived people of the right to choose health care methods.

Despite opposition, doctors and others trained in biomedicine increased their standing within Western society as the 20th century progressed, to the point where, economically, socially, and even politically, they formed an elite group. The alternatives to biomedicine never disappeared, of course. Dominant positions are usually contested, and medical pluralism is still with us. Some current movements, such as holistic health, revive practices that were present in the 19th century and earlier. So, now as always, ideas and practices vie for the attention of consumers in the American medical marketplace. Perhaps, in some respects, nothing much has changed. It is our principal contention in this book, however, that the disillusionment with biomedicine has, over the past few decades, become widespread. There definitely has been a renewal of interest in alternative therapies. In the next section of this chapter, the recent upsurge in alternative use is documented.

THE MAGNITUDE OF THE TREND TOWARD ALTERNATIVE THERAPIES

Evidence has been accumulating for some time indicating that Americans have been turning in increasing numbers to alternative therapies. Documentation of this movement came in 1993, when the prestigious *New England Journal of Medicine* published the results of a national survey. The survey questionnaire asked people if, among other things, they had used one or more of a list of 16 unconventional therapies for a serious or bothersome medical condition in the 12 months prior to the interview (Eisenberg et al., 1993). Despite some methodological shortcomings of the study (which are addressed by Hyatt and Hale in chapter 9), the findings were revealing. One third of the respondents reported using at least one unconventional therapy (e.g., a homeopathic remedy), and of these, one third sought unconventional therapy from a provider.

Contrary to what many of us might have expected, users of unconventional practices were not primarily deprived members of society, those often denied full access to biomedical care. Rather, the highest use was reported by non-Blacks between the ages of 25 and 49 who had relatively high incomes and levels of education. As one might expect, alternative help was sought more for chronic than for life-threatening conditions. Most people (83%) who used an unconventional therapy also sought treatment for the same problem from a medical doctor, reinforcing the ideas of pluralism and pragmatism discussed above.

Eisenberg and his colleagues (1993) used their findings to estimate that in 1990 Americans made 425 million visits to practitioners of unconventional therapies, exceeding the number of visits to all primary care physicians (388 million). Also, people spent approximately $13.7 billion on unconventional therapies. Three fourths of that amount, $10.3 billion, was out-of-pocket, somewhat less than what was spent out-of-pocket for all hospitalizations ($12.8 billion). The article concludes that alternative therapies are being used more than previously reported, that physicians should ask their patients if they are using such therapies, and also that medical students should be taught about unconventional medicine.

Aside from these basic data on alternative health care utilization, some other developments are noteworthy. The federal government clearly has taken a positive interest, albeit rather small, in alternative medicine. Former president Bush signed a bill in 1991 giving the National Institutes of Health (NIH) a $2 million appropriation to evaluate, scientifically, treatments that are not mainstream medical science. The much publicized NIH Office of Alternative Medicine began with a budget of $3.5 million for 1994; it was increased to $7.5 million in fiscal year 1996, and with the addition of aid from other NIH institutes, the grants totaled nearly $10 million. Since the fall of 1995, the office has awarded 3-year grants of about $1 million each to 10 medical centers. The American Public Health Association (APHA) has created a special primary interest group (SPIG) on alternative and complementary health practices, whose members can be both practitioners and researchers. And a group of over 200 alternative practitioners and researchers from throughout the United States submitted a report entitled *Alternative Medicine: Expanding Medical Horizons* (NIH, 1994).

Additionally, there are 17 other Public Health Service agencies providing approximately $12 million for 56 studies on alternative techniques, including the following: the National Institute on Drug Abuse is funding a study on acupuncture for cocaine abuse; the National Institute of Allergy and Infectious Diseases is testing possible anti-HIV compounds found in plants; and the Agency for Health Care Policy and Research is examining chiropractic versus physical therapy for back pain. These activities reflect an evolution in mind-set, at least as some biomedical practitioners and administrators demonstrate.

The fact that scientific research is being conducted that examines the efficacy of therapeutic alternatives to biomedicine should prove of benefit to the public in general, as well as provide legitimacy in specific cases. For example, the field of psychoneuroimmunology has emerged to examine reports of cures from religious shrines, faith healers, shamans, or the laying on of hands. We know that the nervous system influences the immune function, and research in psychopharmacology has brought to light how the brain promotes self-healing (Kearney & Rosch, 1985). Recent research shows that the dichotomy between mind and body, which biomedicine often fostered, is a false dichotomy.

The research just mentioned is being conducted in the natural sciences. Also important is research being carried out in the social sciences. Social scientists have begun to paint multidimensional portraits of alternative therapies and healers, pointing out the strengths and weaknesses of each and looking at the whole alternative movement in terms of its social, cultural, and historical context (Gevitz, 1988).

Recognition of the emerging importance of alternative health therapies is also seen in other, publicly visible ways. A textbook for training clinicians on the fundamentals of complementary and alternative medicine was recently published (Micozzi, 1996). The journalist Bill Moyers (1995) produced a highly acclaimed television series on alternative health practices, along with a companion book, *Healing and the Mind.* Dan Rather, prominent TV newsman, presented a week of special reports on alternative health care. The Australian Broadcasting Corporation produced a series on alternative medicine called *Healers, Quacks or Mystics,* and published a companion book (Drury, 1983). Meredith McGuire, in her book titled *Ritual Healing in Suburban America* (1988), identified more than 130 different types of alternative healers and healing groups that had some following among respondents in the middle-class, suburban portion of a populous northern New Jersey county.

Alternative therapies are penetrating American health care and American society in general in a variety of ways. There are increasing numbers of providers of alternative health care, including those trained in biomedicine. For example, almost 3,000 medical doctors now employ acupuncture in their practice, whereas fewer than 500 did a decade ago. Online computer networks provide a means to readily access holistic and alternative health information. Insurance is covering the services of some alternative health therapies to a greater degree than ever before.[1] Even the Internal Revenue Service accepts expenses for Navajo medicine men, acupuncture, and chiropractic as legitimate medical deductions. The Wellness Network, established by the American Western Life Insurance Company, is a holistically oriented managed care health plan, and Tru-Care, Inc., a preferred provider organization (PPO), is establishing an alternative medicine network (McLaughlin, 1995).

To this point we have focused on the new mind-set in the United States. This is not the only country experiencing a trend toward alternative medicine, however. In Britain, for example, the change is well documented (Jenkins, 1993; Jones, 1995). Use of alternative practices is being advocated increasingly by health ministers, patients, and managers in the National Health Service, who find that they can save money by providing drug-free

---

[1] A chart developed by Goodwin (1997) shows insurance coverage by company, alternative therapies covered, in the state available, and contact telephone number.

treatments. Along with Americans, Britons have become more disillusioned with exclusive reliance on biomedicine and more interested in health matters in general. The British Medical Association has relaxed its former outright hostility to alternative medicine. Now, three fourths of its members refer patients for alternative treatments. Meanwhile, the government has funded a scheme to set national standards for alternative practitioners, and 17 therapies have been identified as meriting registration. Eighty percent of medical students in Britain say that they would like to have training in one or more alternative therapies. Monitoring the British experience can prove fruitful for the United States, as patients, providers, insurance and managed care companies, educators in the health professions, and federal and state policymakers attempt to deal with the increasing popularity of alternative therapies.

PURPOSE: WHAT THIS BOOK ATTEMPTS TO DO

In this chapter we have raised a number of questions. Because health is complex and is affected by a myriad of factors, an interdisciplinary team of scholars from the social sciences, policy sciences, public health, health administration, and nursing and medical professions have written chapters based on their research and professional experience to address the basic questions posed.

Definitive answers are not expected, particularly in such a newly emerging and often controversial field. The purpose of the book is to provide a discussion of salient issues in alternative medicine to a wide audience: consumers, students in the health professions and in health-related courses of other disciplines, practitioners of biomedicine and alternative medicine, administrators of hospitals and health centers, executives of health insurance companies and managed care organizations, managers in the natural and health products industry, and policymakers at all levels of government.

This book can serve as a primer for the neophyte in the field or can provide new insights for those familiar with alternative medicine. People are using alternative therapies regardless of official or professional sanctions. The focus of this book is on the reasons for and the ramifications of increasing utilization, not the efficacy of alternative therapies. If we, the editors and authors, are successful in achieving our goal, readers will come away more aware of and knowledgeable about historical, political, legal, economic, social, and cultural elements, as well as some medical, nursing education, and clinical aspects, of the increasing use of alternative therapies. With this background, readers also will be able to raise their own pertinent questions when faced with the many choices in the increasingly complex health care marketplace.

ORGANIZATION

The book is divided into five parts, incorporating 15 chapters. Part One presents an introduction, history, and framework for understanding what follows; Part Two focuses on politics and the law; Part Three, on the changing medical marketplace; Part Four, on the culture complex; and Part Five, on educational and clinical encounters in complementary medicine. Highlights of chapters within each part are introduced and discussed in terms of how they link to each other and to the major themes of the book. Chapters begin with a general introduction of the topic, followed by specific examples from the authors' research—much of it published for the first time in this book—and conclude with an analysis of trends for the future. Case studies, examples, quotations, and/or vignettes will appear throughout the book to personalize topics. The different approaches illustrate how alternative health care relates to everyday life.

2

The Definitional Dilemma of Alternative Medicine

Barbara Cable Nienstedt

*The significant problems we have cannot be solved
at the same level of thinking we were at
when we created them.*
—*Albert Einstein*

WHAT *IS* ALTERNATIVE MEDICINE?

The phenomenon of alternative medicine as a consumer-driven force in the medical arena has been largely unorganized. This lack of organization has resulted in a need for definitional clarity as to *what* it really is and *who* is included in the vague area known as alternative health. Consistency of definition is a problem in trying to compare within or between biomedicine and alternative categories when the definition of what constitutes *alternative* changes from study to study (as shown in Tables 2.1 and 2.2).

Even the rubric "alternative" medicine itself is questionable, and some prefer other terms such as holistic, complementary, unorthodox, unconventional, natural, traditional, or nontraditional, depending on whose viewpoint is represented. The World Health Organization, for example, considers traditional medicine to be the indigenous folk medicine of countries; their definition of biomedicine is known as conventional medicine. In contrast, biomedicine in our country is often considered traditional medicine, and forms different from this are called alternative.

As a starting point to resolve some of the confusion, we suggest use of the term *alternative* as a generic category to describe all therapies and practices outside the predominant biomedical profession. This seems to be the

TABLE 2.1   Examples of Alternative Medicine Definitions in Previous Research

Author	Definitions
Fairfoot (1987, p. 384)	Those treatment modalities which stem from beliefs about the nature and causation of disease which are at variance with and indeed antagonistic to, contemporary orthodox knowledge and practice.
Corry (1983, p. 13)	If . . . alternative practitioners have anything in common, it is an opposition to traditional [Western] medicine and possibly to the constraints inherent in the scientific method and professional codes of ethics.
Fulder (1986, p. 236)	Alternative medicine . . . encompasses a variety of therapeutic systems which are joined by the fact that they are different from conventional medicine.
McGuire (1988, p. 3)	A wide range of beliefs and practices that adherents expect to affect health but that are not promulgated by the medical personnel in the dominant biomedical system.
Murray & Rubel (1992, p. 61)	A heterogeneous set of practices that are offered as an alternative to conventional medicine for the preservation of health and the diagnosis and treatment of health-related problems.
Fugh-Berman (1993, p. 241)	The term "alternative medicine" is maddeningly broad, encompassing as it does complete ancient medical systems such as *ayurvedic* and traditional Chinese medicine as well as single component (and sometimes single proponent) regimens such as bee pollen or ozone therapies.
Eisenberg et al. (1993, p. 246)	Medical practices that are not in conformity with the standards of the medical community.

From Osborn, 1997.

most generally accepted term by a majority of professionals, both biomedical and alternative, and by the public. We use the term *complementary medicine* to describe the cooperative effort between biomedicine and alternative practitioners in pursuit of their patients' good health and well-being. *Holistic* will be used to describe concepts or therapies based on the principles of prevention of disease and the interconnectedness, or wholeness, of all aspects of the patient (mental, physical, and spiritual). As Weil (1988) notes, "Holistic medicine is an informal collection of attitudes and practices, not a defined system of treatment" (p. 181). Holistic concepts are primarily

TABLE 2.2 Examples of Categorizations of Alternative Medicine in Previous Research

Authors	No. of Categories	Types of Alternative Healers
Gardner (1957, pp. 186–203)	4	Chiropractic, homeopathy, naturopathy, osteopathy
Corry (1983, pp. 82–105)	5	Scientific basis: biofeedback and autogenics, clinical ecology, holistic health, homeopathy, guided imagery
	12	No scientific basis: acupuncture, aura healing, chiropractic, Christian Science, faith healing, naturopathy, negative ion therapy, orthomolecular therapy, psychic surgery, pyramid power, Scientology, voodoo
Achterberg (1988, pp. 74–75)	8	Ayurvedic, behavioral medicine, Chinese medicine, chiropractic, holistic medicine, homeopathy, metaphysical and esoteric healing, Native American medicine
Gevitz (1988)	8	Chiropractic, Christian Science, contemporary folk medicine, divine healing, homeopathy, hydropathy, nineteenth century botanical medicine, osteopathy
Knipschild et al. (1990)	6	Acupuncture, homeopathy, spiritual techniques, manual therapies, natural remedies, orthomolecular medicine, miscellaneous therapies
Eisenberg et al. (1993)	18	Acupuncture, biofeedback, chiropractic, commercial weight loss programs, energy healing, exercise, folk remedies, herbal medicine, homeopathy, hypnosis, imagery, lifestyle diets, massage, megavitamin therapy, prayer, relaxation techniques, self-help groups, spiritual healing

From Osborn, 1997.

used by alternative practitioners, but a small number of biomedicine practitioners also adhere to holistic principles. These basic definitions are important for purposes of consistency within our book.

A thornier definitional issue emerges when trying to refine the vast number of practices residing within the alternative category to better understand if or how they fit together. McGuire, in her book *Ritual Healing in Suburban America* (1988), identified over 130 different healing groups and individuals used by suburban residents of a single county in New Jersey. This large number illustrates the need for categorization to better comprehend the diversity and sometimes bewildering categories of alternative medicine.

Over the years researchers have attempted to codify the healing practices of alternative medicine. Generally, there is little agreement as to which practices constitute this group. The Office of Alternative Medicine (OAM) (National Institutes of Health, 1994) created seven categories of alternative medical practices:

- Diet/nutrition/lifestyle changes
- Mind/body interventions
- Alternative systems
- Bioelectromagnetic applications in medicine
- Manual healing methods
- Pharmacological and biological treatments
- Herbal medicine

The OAM notes that the classification was designed to facilitate their grant process and should not be considered definitive. While acknowledging the difficulty of categorization, we nonetheless find these classifications are not very informative outside that stated purpose of grant review. For example, in the OAM model, depending on one's definition, massage therapy might fit under manual healing methods, alternative systems, mind/body interventions, or herbal medicine (if herbs are used externally). Does faith healing fall into lifestyle changes, mind/body interventions, or alternative systems? Consensus on which categories to place even these two rather simple examples in is lacking.

Gordon and Nienstedt (1992) presented a more parsimonious model of complementary medicine, based on four quadrants that helped them to introduce some order into the discussion of numerous and varied health care practices. The four quadrants represent groups of biomedical practitioners, body healing alternative practitioners, mind/spirit alternative practitioners, and cross-cultural alternative practitioners. They acknowledged that such an approach, while desirable and enlightening, also has its limitations. As seen above with the OAM model, therapies do not always fit neatly into exclusive categories. Moreover, as interactions among all sectors increase (a goal well worth pursuing), the distinctive lines between the practices may blur even more.

Figure 2.1 illustrates a model that is based on the different healing philosophies of alternative and biomedicine practitioners and is proposed to inform the discussion of complementary medical practices. There may be some crossover among the model segments in terms of therapeutic practices, but the model nonetheless serves to initiate and inform the discussion of complementary medical practices. Figure 2.1 also provides examples of some of the practices belonging in each of these segments.

The model is divided into quadrants based on the patient-consumers who use these healing practices. Alternative medicine occupies three quadrants of the model, not because of numerical preponderance, as the numbers are largely unknown, but because of its diversity in approach. The model's four quadrants are represented as follows:

Biomedicine is the quadrant in the model most familiar to the general public. It represents the predominant biomedicine medical paradigm. Physicians and nurses are practitioners who primarily focus their treatment on the patient-consumer's disease and its cure. It is an approach that identifies and isolates the problem area and directs surgery, pharmaceutical remedies, and sophisticated technology to its treatment and cure. The following professions are among those occupying the Biomedicine quadrant:

- Chiropodists
- Dentists
- Dental hygienists
- Dietitians
- Emergency medical technicians
- Medical doctors
- Medical technologists
- Nurses (including nurse practitioners and nurse midwives)
- Optometrists
- Osteopathic doctors
- Pharmacists
- Physical therapists
- Physician assistants
- Psychologists
- Podiatrists
- Radiological technologists
- Respiratory therapists

Alternative medicine practices can be viewed in three quadrants of the model. We understand the holistic approach to healing involves the interconnectedness of mind, body, and spirit, but it is helpful to refine our understanding by differentiating those therapies that approach healing from a primary emphasis on body, mind/spirit, or cross-cultural aspects.

Body Healing Alternatives is the terminology used for the next quadrant. As in most alternative health philosophies, practitioners believe in the integrative connection of the whole person (i.e., a holistic view) as opposed to

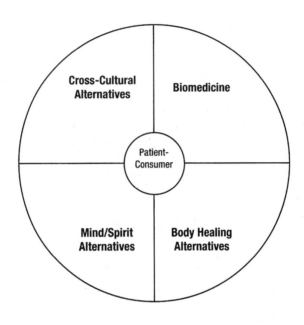

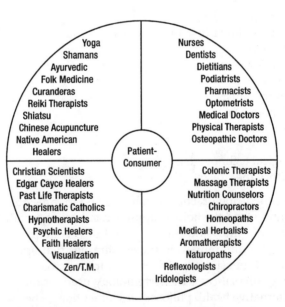

FIGURE 2.1 Models of complementary medicine and practice.

the localized disease perspective (an allopathic view) of biomedicine. Alternative medical treatments in this quadrant focus on internal and/or external body work. For purposes of easier classification and understanding, we list the following practices in the Body Healing quadrant separately, as having primarily an external or an internal approach (see Table 2.3). We recognize, however, that these approaches are often not exclusive of one another and, given individual needs, that the emphasis may vary.

Mind/spirit alternatives encompass religious, spiritual, and metaphysical treatment. Practitioners believe the mind or spirit is the vehicle for controlling and, therefore, healing the body through prayer, altered levels of consciousness, or visualization. Examples in the mind/spirit quadrant are as follows:

- Art therapy
- Autogenic therapy
- Charismatic Catholics
- Christian Science
- Color therapy
- Edgar Cayce remedies
- Faith healers
- Guided imagery/visualization
- Humor therapy
- Hypnotherapy
- Meditation
- Music, sound therapy
- Past life/regression therapy
- Psychic healers
- Psychotherapy

Cross-cultural alternatives are approaches to healing that may have existed on the American continent for centuries, as Native American, Southern Appalachian, African American, Afro-Caribbean, and Mexican American, or they may have been carried more recently from cultures in other countries of the world. They are currently being accepted by some of the public as viable treatment alternatives. Treatments vary, and some are based on complicated systems of medicine developed thousands of years before biomedicine. Ayurvedic and Chinese medicine, for example, are ancient in origin and hold that a person is an integrated system in which the observed symptoms of a disease are actually the result of a dysfunction elsewhere in the body. Therefore, cancer of the breast may be viewed as originating from an imbalance in the liver. Treatment would consequently be directed at the liver. Additionally, cross-cultural approaches take the holistic view of the person, considering both the body *and* mind/spirit aspects.

TABLE 2.3   Examples of Body Healing Alternatives

Primarily external approaches

Alexander technique	Magnetic field therapy
Applied kinesiology	Metabolic therapy
Aston patterning	Myotherapy
Biofeedback	Neural therapy
Body energy therapies	Oxidizing agents therapy
Bodywork therapies	Oxygen therapy
Chiropractic	Polarity therapy
Cranial sacral therapy	Reconstructive therapy
Ear coning therapy	Reflexology
Electromagnetic therapy	Reiki massage
Energy medicine	Rolfing
Environmental medicine	Rosen methods
Feldenkrais methods	Schuessler tissue salts
Hellerwork	Therapeutic massage
Hydrotherapy and hyperthermia	Therapeutic touch
Iridology	Trager method
Lepore technique	Zone therapy
Light therapy	

Primarily internal approaches

Applied nutrition	Enzyme therapy
Antineoplaston therapy	Fasting therapies
Aromatherapy	Herbal medicine
Bach flower remedies	Homeopathy
Cell therapy (antineoplastins)	Juice therapy
Chelation therapy	Macrobiotics
Colon therapy	Naturopathy
Detoxification therapy	Orthomolecular medicine

As noted by Crellin (1987), the health care scene is a particularly fruitful one in which to pose general questions about cultural interactions and transmission of belief. Why do some healing beliefs persist longer than others? Crellin's view is that, for the maintenance of these beliefs, reinforcement is necessary from one generation to the next. Moreover, he states that "popular beliefs—unacceptable to modern medical science—are more widespread than is commonly thought. Certainly they contribute to the feeling that physicians and pharmacists have become more impersonal in recent decades and out-of-touch with many patients" (p. 117). The following are examples in the Cross-Cultural quadrant:

- Acupuncture and acupressure
- Ayurvedic medicine

- *Chi gong* or *qigong*
- *Curanderismo*
- Folk medicine
- *Jin shin jyutsu*
- Moxibustion
- Native American medicine men/women
- *Reiki*
- Shamanism
- Shiatsu
- Tai chi
- Traditional Chinese medicine
- Voodoo
- Witch doctors
- Yoga

The above examples are intended to be as exhaustive as possible, but it is evident from the rich diversity of alternative practitioners and the dynamic nature of some of the therapies that this may fall somewhat short of the mark. As new alternative practices surface, they may be added to these descriptive categories of body healing, mind/spirit, and cross-cultural.

A few problematic cases surfaced immediately and required judgment calls as to which quadrant of the model was most appropriate. The most obvious was the profession of osteopathy. In the beginning its healing practices were based on true alternative methods of prevention and holistic health. As surgery and pharmaceutical interventions were added, the perspective changed to reflect more of the predominant biomedical approach, focusing these interventions on the disease and its cure. Presently, a case could be made for them to be placed in either biomedicine or alternative systems. We have arguably placed them in the biomedical because their emphasis on drugs, hospitals, and surgery appears more in line with the thinking of that model. Homeopaths, as a second example, are required to be medical doctors in some states but not in others. For that reason they are included in the alternative category, but this is also admittedly debatable for those homeopaths who are licensed medical doctors. A final example is illustrated in the case of midwives. Because of their different orientations, nurse midwives belong in the Biomedicine quadrant, but folk or "granny" midwives are more accurately placed in the Alternative quadrant. We have placed midwives as a practice in the Biomedical quadrant; folk midwives are then considered as part of folk medicine practices in the Alternative quadrant. Despite these three examples, the model tends to work quite well in a descriptive and parsimonious sense for most other practices.

WHO *ARE* THESE ALTERNATIVE PRACTITIONERS?

In a glossary compiled by the author, which can be found at the end of this book, descriptions of alternative health practices are offered. Because of the dynamic nature of their presence in the healing arena, the glossary focuses on practices currently in use. Undertaking the listing of practitioners and therapists in alternative health care is an arduous but necessary task. First, it serves to illustrate the rationale behind choosing placement in the model categories. Second, describing these alternative approaches in a succinct few sentences certainly does not do justice to the depth of their philosophy or practice, but it does serve to acquaint the reader with a sense of the variety and large numbers of alternative practices and the basic similarities or differences among therapies. Just as with biomedical practices, some of these alternatives are here to stay, others pass through, fall into disuse, and occasionally resurface decades or centuries later.

An intriguing example of a widespread alternative practice that has largely fallen into disuse is Fletcherism, a theory of the early 1900s that was based on disease being caused by indigestion or poor assimilation of food. Proper chewing, which was central to this theory, came to be known as "Fletcherizing," and Horace Fletcher himself was known as the Great Masticator. A 1914 article in the *Ladies' Home Journal* admonished "Don't gobble your food, but 'Fletcherize.'" Fletcher was favorably received by such academic giants as Cambridge, Harvard, and Yale. His books were translated into several languages, and serious articles about him appeared in respected journals such as the British medical journal *Lancet* (Armstrong & Armstrong, 1991). Reflecting on what seems like a ludicrous practice from our present-day perspective, we must keep in mind that the biomedical cures of those same days required purging a patient of disease through bleeding and vomiting and applications of leeches. Although playing a considerably reduced role today, thorough mastication remains a component of several alternative practices.

An aspect of alternative medical practices that is frequently overlooked is the complexity of many of the belief systems in this area. When the typical biomedical practitioner and patient are first exposed to alternative medical practices, they sometimes come to know them on a superficial level, not understanding the underlying philosophies, connections, and principles of the healing system involved. From that perspective, the practices may seem ludicrous, unsophisticated, and unscientific. It should be noted, though, that taken out of context and without a depth of understanding, even biomedical techniques can appear bizarre and counterintuitive.

Using traditional Chinese medicine as an example, we note several profound concepts that compose a complete and complicated system of medicine that has existed for millennia. Just as it is possible for lay persons to administer first aid effectively, it is also possible for Westerners to learn and even practice certain aspects of Chinese medicine. But it is done without knowing or understanding the Chinese system's complex underlying foundation and theories. Essential concepts such as *yin* and *yang* (pronounced *yahng)*; the five elemental phases—fire, water, earth, metal, and wood; and a wide range of personal and environmental factors must be understood and mastered before truly practicing Chinese traditional medicine. In a similar vein, training to become a medicine man in the Native American healing system takes longer than training to become a surgeon. Labeling these cultural practices and other alternative therapies as "unscientific" often belies an ignorance of the depth and complexity of the practice.

An unfortunate example of this lack of understanding is found in the *New Wellness Encyclopedia* (Editors, 1995) written by the editors of the University of California–Berkeley Wellness Letter. They dismiss macrobiotic diets as "nutritional quackery," noting, without providing a citation, "you are eventually supposed to cut out all foods except brown rice" (p. 25). In reading several books on macrobiotic diet and way of life, I found no evidence advocating that practice. Indeed, the macrobiotic diet includes whole grains with fresh vegetables, sea vegetables, and fruits in a complex balancing of yin and yang energy, along with the consideration of individual and environmental factors for both prevention and healing of disease.

CONCLUSIONS

The definitional dilemmas of what and who are alternative health practitioners may be slowly moving toward consensus. The more pejorative rubrics of unorthodox and unconventional are fading from use, and the more value-neutral one of alternative is being used more consistently. It should be noted, however, that some authors and practitioners feel that *alternative* has negative connotations as well and prefer the term *holistic* to describe nonbiomedical practices. Our view is that holistic concepts will be increasingly added to biomedical practices of the future, causing definitional confusion. The term *alternative medicine* as a body of nonbiomedical practices seems a better description to us.

Definitive listings and categorization of alternative practices may be slower to form consensus. The field is so dynamic that slight modifications to existing therapies result in several different therapeutic names, some of which are used by only a small number of devotees. Categorizations such as the model proposed in this chapter makes it easier to grasp the fundamental focus of the practices even when they overlap. Once typologies achieve consensus and are used more regularly, research efforts can become more methodical and comparisons become easier and more consistent.

Resolution of the definitional dilemmas is followed by another problem area, which may prove more resistant. Aspects of the spiritual, physical, mental, and emotional dimensions are increasingly being incorporated into today's healing practices. Many of these healing practices take time and study to understand the philosophies behind the practices and to appreciate the complexity of the healing system on which they are built, but that also makes them more coherent and logical. Also, the global interconnectedness of the past decade demands sensitivity to cross-cultural healing therapies as well. The level of profundity required for understanding systems used by Chinese or Ayurvedic practitioners, for example, is daunting. In the case of the University of California–Berkeley editors mentioned above, cultural sensitivity to the foundations of many Eastern healing philosophies would have given them a greater understanding of the macrobiotic diet, even the practice of eating only brown rice. For several thousand years, religious ascetics have used healing practices that require extreme diets or fasts to achieve spiritual predominance over their physical bodies in order for healing to occur. These diets and fasts have been (and continue to be) used by people of many cultures and faiths, including, perhaps, some macrobiotic ascetics.

As alternative therapies grow in strength and numbers, our knowledge of the diversity of available choices must expand as well. Patients are now, more than ever before, participating *consumers* in their health care decisions, with a wide variety of economic and philosophical choices.

PART II

Politics and the Law

*The health of the people is really the foundation upon which
all their happiness and all their powers as a state depend.*
—*Benjamin Disraeli, 1887*

The three chapters in this section examine the idea that the position of alternative medicine vis à vis biomedicine is strongly influenced by politics, powerful economic interests, and the legal system. In chapter 3, Barbara Cable Nienstedt discusses three possible outcomes stemming from these influences. The first outcome is co-optation or the official recognition of alternative practices; perhaps the best example of this is the incorporation of osteopathy within biomedicine in the United States. The second possible outcome is "quackbusting," or enforcing regulations that curb certain alternative practices in the name of protecting the public. The attempts by the American Medical Association to eliminate chiropractic in the United States is a prime example here. The third possible outcome is that alternative medicine and biomedicine will be truly complementary, separate but equal.

In chapter 4, Leonard Baer and Charles Good examine laws and policies within and among states to ascertain how the power of the state influences the location and mobility of alternative providers. Acupuncture, chiropractic, and homeopathy are given as major examples of the variation of provider practice acts among states in 1995. The authors note that having or not having a state practice act does not necessarily mean that a practice is illegal. For example, some states that permit non-MD acupuncture or require training for MD acupuncturists do so despite the absence of a practice act.

Kristen Borré and James Wilson show, in chapter 5, how two professionalized medical paradigms, homeopathy and biomedicine, clashed in the United States. Tracing the history of this conflict, they describe how homeopathy went from a position of equality and even some dominance in the 19th century to extreme marginalization as an alternative practice because of strong allopathic opposition and various historical circumstances.

Currently, however, homeopathy is finding increasing acceptance, especially in the treatment of chronic illness. Several aspects of homeopathy are
described, including the theory of how and why it works, what research
has been done, how practitioners are trained, how services are delivered
(with examples from North Carolina and Pennsylvania), the pharmaceutical and treatment materials support system, issues of legal and economic
regulation, and public expectations. They suggest that homeopathy and
biomedicine can and should be used in complementary ways to make a
more effective overall health care system.

3

The Federal Approach to Alternative Medicine: Co-opting, Quackbusting, or Complementing?

Barbara Cable Nienstedt

> *To restrict the art of healing to one class of men*
> *and deny equal privileges to others will constitute the Bastille*
> *of medical science. The Constitution of this republic should make*
> *special privilege for medical freedom as well as religious freedom.*
> —*Benjamin Rush, MD, signer of the Declaration of Independence*

POLITICAL AND LEGAL BATTLES

In the early years of the United States there was a multiplicity of medical practitioners and health practices operating with virtually no government regulation or professional restrictions. The popular health movement, inspired by Andrew Jackson's sentiment of antielitism, led to the end of almost all government regulation of health care. By 1845, Jacksonian efforts left only three states still licensing medical doctors, thereby encouraging availability of a wide variety of competitive practices. By the end of the 19th century, though, the contest had narrowed considerably (Coulter, 1982). Powerful political alliances, professional lobbying organizations, and abundant use of the courts were necessary for the rise to preeminence of allopathic medicine.

An important effort in ensuring that standards were based on the biomedical model came about early in the 20th century. Abraham Flexner (1910) produced a report on the status of medical education in the United

States and Canada. Based on allopathic standards and sponsored by the Carnegie Foundation, the Flexner report was a devastating critique of medical schools. This public exposure, combined with gradually stricter state licensing laws, forced many medical schools of all orientations to close their doors or ally themselves with recognized universities. Although the quality of medical education improved as a result of the report, of more political importance was the fact that the improvement weeded out many disciplines having smaller numbers. The economic burden of compliance for these schools could not be supported by tuition or financial support from established universities. Allopathic educational standards consequently became the exclusionary yardstick by which all health care professions would be measured.

CO-OPTING: OFFICIAL RECOGNITION

Gaining official or professional acceptance has always been the supreme challenge for alternative medicine in this century. One of the easiest ways to become accepted is to join the ranks of the established profession. Adopting the theory and practice of the predominant group, which often requires abandoning your own theory and practice, is essential for inclusion.

One example of this co-optation is found in the history of the osteopathic profession. Although its founder, Andrew Taylor Still, was a medical doctor, he broke with mainstream medicine and founded a new system based on the "rule of the artery." Healthy arteries, Still said, constricted by spinal displacements, disturbed the blood's circulation and induced disease. Osteopaths treated disease by manipulating the tissues of the body, especially those that support the backbone and the nerves between the vertebrae. In 1892, Still founded the first osteopathic school of medicine in Missouri (Armstrong & Armstrong, 1991).

As state regulation of medical schools increased, osteopaths spent less time on spinal manipulation and were forced to add once-forbidden surgery and pharmacology classes in order to comply with state standards. Graduates of the new classes were derisively called "three-fingered osteopaths" by their older colleagues, who used both hands for spinal adjustments—three fingers being all that was required to write out a drug prescription. Goaded by the Flexner report, osteopathic colleges were also forced to tighten entrance requirements and lengthen the time to graduation to meet new standards. In a shrewd political countermove, the American Osteopathic Association was formed in 1901; modeled after the American Medical Association (AMA), it produced a journal and began AMA-style lobbying to liberalize state licensing. The members were enormously successful in getting all 50 states to legalize osteopathy by 1974, giving them the same rights as MDs.

Perhaps the most unusual example of biomedical co-optation can be seen in California's experience with osteopaths. In 1962 osteopathic doctors were given the opportunity of converting their DO degrees to MDs. Two thousand of the state's 2,300 osteopaths accepted the offer in return for giving up their status (and beliefs) as osteopaths. MDs generally saw the benefit of this absorption approach—it enlarged their political base and freed them from expending energy fighting osteopaths on a professional front. In addition, Armstrong and Armstrong (1991) note that the merger removed California osteopaths, the country's most dynamic and academically gifted, from the ranks of competition with MDs.

CONGRESSIONAL ACTION

Federal recognition of alternative medicine came from Congress, probably in response to public pressures from advocates and users of alternative medicine. The National Institutes of Health (NIH) received an appropriation from Congress in 1991 for purposes of open meetings and public hearings on "unconventional medical practices." They convened a working group of individuals and organizations interested in research and validation of unconventional or alternative medical practices. As noted in the *Federal Register* (Office of Science Policy and Legislation, 1992), this working group would then participate in a planning workshop, to be held several months later, designed to further evaluation efforts of unconventional medicine. Central to the agenda of both meetings was, first, the identification of the alternative medical community and, second, the identification of barriers to evaluating the effectiveness of alternative medical practices. At this workshop, 10 working groups identified and classified seven categories of alternative medical practices:

- Diet/nutrition/lifestyle changes
- Mind/body interventions
- Alternative systems
- Bioelectromagnetic applications
- Manual healing methods
- Pharmacological and biological treatments
- Herbal medicine

The working groups later issued a report on the status of alternative medicine in the United States (National Institutes of Health, 1994) and noted some of the barriers to evaluating effectiveness, among which were research methodology and the peer review process.

THE OFFICE OF ALTERNATIVE MEDICINE

The original name of the office, Unconventional Medical Practices, accurately reflected its general position in the medical hierarchy. After 2 years as an interim office in NIH, it became codified in June 1993. Many alternative health practitioners objected to the term *unconventional* because they felt it carried a pejorative connotation of being on the fringe of medical respectability. A name change followed, and the Office of Alternative Medicine (OAM) was officially recognized by the federal establishment. The Congressional mandate stated that the purpose of establishing an office for unconventional medical practices was to facilitate evaluation of the effectiveness of alternative treatments and to help integrate effective treatments into the medical mainstream. In addition, the OAM was to act as a clearinghouse for information and data on alternative health. A Program Advisory Council was set up in 1994; 18 members meet three times a year to provide advice to the OAM director.

Currently, OAM activities are focused on sponsoring research, encouraging the biomedical paradigm with "collaboration between *orthodox* [italics added] research investigators and alternative [the implied contrast is unorthodox] medical practitioners." The office also conducts conferences, along with grant writing and clinical research workshops teaching *biomedical* protocols. Two exploratory centers for alternative medical research have been funded in 1994 for $1.68 million over a 3-year period. Bastyr University in Seattle, Washington, is examining alternative treatments for HIV/ AIDS; Minneapolis Medical Research Foundation is evaluating addictions and related disorders.

A major function of the OAM is cooperation and collaboration with the appropriate organizations within the NIH. Networking with the Food and Drug Administration (FDA), Health Care Financing Agency (HCFA), Agency for Health Care Policy and Research (AHCPR), and other large mainstream agencies is strongly encouraged, including regular meetings with the FDA "to enroll its cooperation in reevaluating the interpretation of current rules and regulations governing research on and use of devices, herbs and homeopathic remedies" (General Information Package, June 1995).

"QUACKBUSTING": THE POLITICS OF ENFORCEMENT

Each branch of the federal government is involved in the political and legal progress (or lack of progress) of alternative medicine's accessibility to the public. The purpose of many government entities in regard to alternative medicine is often stated as the protection of the public from harmful or ineffective substances and practices. Powerful and heavily financed lobbies of interested biomedical organizations also bring pressure to bear on the government in an effort to limit that accessibility, often by questioning the competence and motives of nonallopathic practitioners. The term *quack* is used almost exclusively in the politics of enforcement to label practitioners of alternative medicine. State boards of medical examiners are charged with enforcing biomedical standards to eliminate substandard practice in their own professions, but the enforcement efforts of these boards, as with many trade and professional regulatory boards, are notoriously weak to nonexistent.

Political and legal pressures intensify as economic interests are threatened. The quackbusting attempts experienced by chiropractors in their drive to achieve professional status provides an interesting contrast to the osteopaths' co-optation example above. Instead of trying to join the ranks of the MDs, chiropractors chose to retain their professional identity and fight quackbusting efforts on numerous legal and political fronts. Their primary opponent was the AMA, which used its considerable strength of numbers and dollars to pursue chiropractors through the courts and the public and professional arenas from 1912 through 1987.

Like other institutions, including biomedical schools, chiropractic schools were hit hard by the Flexner report. Additionally, they faced an organized effort to eradicate their profession completely. Antichiropractic articles were published in the official documents of the *Journal of the American Medical Association (JAMA)* beginning in 1912 (Armstrong & Armstrong, 1991), and intense legal and political battles ensued until 1987, when chiropractors won a historic antitrust lawsuit against the AMA.

Over the years since 1912 the AMA has made chiropractic the subject of numerous studies and official positions, from the Committee on the Costs of Medical Care to the Committee on Quackery. Reports called for the containment, if not the elimination, of chiropractic. In an official statement from the AMA House of Delegates, chiropractic was deemed "a hazard to rational health care . . . because of substandard and unscientific education . . . and rigid adherence to an irrational, unscientific approach to disease causation" (AMA, 1966). The AMA considered the discipline a dangerous cult.

Chiropractors were attacked on the legal front as well. From 1906 to 1927 the Universal Chiropractic Association handled 3,300 legal charges. During the first 30 years of the profession's existence more than 15,000 prosecutions were *brought to trial* (Wardwell, 1988). No figures are available on the number of charges that were actually filed against chiropractors but not brought to trial. If the proportions are even remotely close to present ratios, the numbers would be staggering. Chiropractors won their first major legal victory in 1913, when Kansas granted them licenses to practice medicine. Despite heavy lobbying from the AMA, 30 states followed with licensing by 1931. All 50 states gave professional recognition by 1974 (Armstrong & Armstrong, 1991).

The chiropractic profession's most aggressive stand was taken against the AMA in 1976. In *Wilk v. AMA* (1987) five Illinois chiropractors filed a federal antitrust suit against the AMA and nine other medical organizations. Similar suits were filed in New York and Pennsylvania. The AMA quickly backed off from its public criticism of chiropractors, but the legal battle continued. The suit was not settled for 11 more years. A United States district judge found in 1987 (*Wilk v. AMA*, 1987) that the AMA had engaged in a conspiracy to contain and eliminate the chiropractic profession and barred the AMA from restricting, regulating, or impeding its members or the hospitals where its members worked from associating with chiropractors.

THE WEB OF ENFORCEMENT

Since the beginning of this century, alternative medicine has been subject to a complex tangle of federal laws, regulations, and court decisions designed to protect the consumer of medical services and products by restricting access to the marketplace.

FEDERAL LAWS

The first attempts to regulate food and drugs through federal law began shortly after the Civil War. More than 100 bills were introduced into Congress between 1879 and 1905, but most failed through lack of public support (Evers, 1988). The sentiment changed because of a scandal involving canned beef during the Spanish-American War. It was said that the meat was so dangerous that it killed more men than Spanish bullets (Johnson, 1982). The Pure Food and Drug Act of 1906 (Chapter 3915, Sections 1–13, 34 Stat. 768) was the result of this scandal. The 1906 act set standards of purity only for food and drugs in interstate commerce. Manufacturers were required to list the nature and quantity of ingredients, and they were prohibited from adulterating or misbranding their products. It is important to note that there were no provisions for review of safety or efficacy.

Numerous flaws in this law went largely uncorrected until an alleged "wonder drug" (elixir of sulfanilamide) killed nearly 100 people in 1937 because the manufacturer had performed no toxicity tests. The 1906 act was repealed and replaced with the federal Food, Drug and Cosmetic Act (FDCA) of 1938 (21 U.S.C. 301–392). For the first time, manufacturers were prohibited from marketing new drugs until they convinced the FDA that they were safe.

Another tragedy led to amendment of the FDCA. The Kefauver-Harris Drug Amendments of 1962 (PL 87–781, 76 Stat. 780) responded to the thalidomide disaster in Europe, which produced children with deformed limbs. Although the FDA had not yet approved thalidomide for safety, Congress added to the safety requirement and mandated that drugs also be proved *effective* for their intended uses.

The next major revision came when Congress enacted the Medical Devices Amendments of 1976 (PL94-295, 90 Stat. 539). These amendments broadened the scope of regulation to ensure that medical devices, like drugs, be proved safe and effective before their introduction into interstate commerce.

Most recently, fierce debate centered around the Nutritional Labeling Enforcement Act (NLEA) of 1990 (PL 101–535, 104 Stat 2353). Congress originally designed the legislation to better educate consumers by providing them with more information on food and nutritional supplement labels. The FDA was delegated the responsibility for enforcing the act. In doing so, the agency developed rigid standards for health benefit claims and extended their definition of labeling to include product names, symbols, logos, and vignettes. Any suggestions implying health benefits would be strictly forbidden unless they met those rigid standards. Endorsements, even from establishment organizations like the American Heart Association, were not allowed. Dietary supplements and herbs were hit especially hard. The FDA encouraged Congress to pass legislation that would bind the Federal Trade Commission (FTC) to those same standards in their regulation of false advertising. The FTC did not agree and opposed FDA's legislative efforts (Evers, 1988).

Public outrage from the economically burgeoning alternative health community forced a Congressional moratorium on NLEA enforcement in 1992. The moratorium was designed to study further and perhaps cool the political temperature. In 1993 the moratorium expired and was replaced by the Hatch/Richardson Amendments (S. 784 and H.R. 1709) to the FDCA. These amendments became known as the Dietary Supplement Health and Education Act (DSHEA) of 1994 (PL 103–417). The act contained provisions for a broader definition of nutritional supplement to include herbs and other supplements. It also recognized that dietary supplements were not drugs or food additives. Grass-roots lobbying by the alternative health community resulted in brochures, bulletins, meetings, and phone trees urging patients and consumers to petition Congress to pass the bill. The effectiveness of this effort was evident when, in October 1994, President Clinton signed the bipartisan DSHEA into law.

FEDERAL POLICIES

The laws mentioned above are designed to protect the consumer against potential harm from unsafe and ineffective health products in the marketplace. To enforce these laws, Congress delegated broad regulatory power to several federal agencies. Perhaps the most powerful agency for both alternative medicine and biomedicine is the federal Food and Drug Administration (FDA). The FTC, the U.S. Postal Service (USPS), and the U.S. Department of Justice (DOJ) are also major players in this broad area of enforcement.

Food and Drug Administration

Great power was given to the FDA through two important provisions of the FDCA. First, the ability to classify a product as food, drug, or cosmetic has enormous consequences for health products and public accessibility to them. The laws' definitions are so broad that they provide immense latitude to the FDA in making that decision. The food/drug dichotomy is shown through two rather commonplace products. Honey is normally considered food. If, however, honey is promoted as being helpful for certain ailments, the FDA will regulate it as a drug. The same dichotomy applies in the case of bran. Kellogg's All-Bran advertising campaign was based on a review of research and prepared with the advice and cooperation of the National Cancer Institute. The FDA investigated the advertisements after pressure from the American Cancer Society, which protested that the advertisements might be misleading to consumers. Ultimately, the FDA abandoned the probe but drafted new standards for making health claims.

The second important provision of the FDCA states that if a product is designated a drug or medical device it is required to undergo an extensive, time-consuming, and expensive process prior to release in the marketplace. Lengthy laboratory and animal testing are required before manufacturers can petition the FDA for an investigational new drug (IND) application for human testing. Critics, including the AMA, complain that the IND process takes nearly 10 years and costs as much as $250 million. Access to new products (or even *old* products redefined as drugs) is consequently limited only to those drug companies that can afford to go through the costly process (Lazlo, 1987).

Claims of FDA abuse of their considerable power of regulation have been plentiful. In July 1995 the first oversight hearing on the FDA's abuse of power was held by the House Oversight and Investigations Subcommittee of the Commerce Committee. In a unique attempt to reach consumers, they established an e-mail address so that allegations of FDA abuse could be reported directly to the subcommittee. The hearings were to be a prelude to drafting FDA reform legislation. No reform bill has surfaced as of this writing.

Without question, the FDA can point with pride to some of their successful efforts to protect the public, and the agency deserves commendation in those cases. The biomedical establishment has regarded the FDA as an essential tool in the government's efforts to combat "quackery" and fraud for the patient's own good. Of all the enforcement agencies, though, the FDA occupies a special place in the hearts of alternative medical practitioners. Whether justified or not, its enforcement efforts have been singled out as being the most egregious example of government suppression of medical freedoms. Over the years the FDA has vigorously pursued a policy of regulation of nutritional supplements. Dozens of alternative health practitioners have claimed to be victims of FDA overzealousness. One of the loudest rallying cries of alternative health professionals has been raised for Jonathan Wright, MD, an outspoken critic of the FDA policies. On May 6, 1992, the door to Dr. Wright's clinic in Kent, Washington, was broken down and, with a waiting room full of patients, the clinic was raided by FDA agents in full combat gear with guns drawn. Agents confiscated everything from confidential patient files, office furniture, supplies, equipment, and even stamps to vitamins and botanical extracts. Advocates of alternative health care say Dr. Wright was singled out because he has been publicly vocal about his treatment methods. Dr. Wright feels that the raid was tied to his filing a lawsuit against the FDA in federal court over the earlier seizure of his stock of an amino acid. Four years later the FDA has still not filed any charges against him.

In addition to claims of overzealous enforcement, critics of the agency cite its most offensive behaviors: blatant ties to the pharmaceutical industry and arbitrary regulation of nutritional supplements and herbs. One study found that half of high-ranking FDA officials were formerly key executives in pharmaceutical companies prior to joining the FDA. Moreover, half of these FDA officials would then go to pharmaceutical companies on leaving the FDA (Lynes, 1992). Using data from the nation's poison control centers, Julian Whitaker notes that only one death occurred from overuse of a supplement in the period from 1983 to 1990. Government data show, however, that there are approximately 130,000 deaths a year from drug use in hospitalized patients (Burton Goldberg Group, 1995, p. 23).

Federal Trade Commission

The FTC statutes contain both a general prohibition of unfair or deceptive acts affecting commerce and a specific provision prohibiting false advertising of food, drugs, devices, or cosmetics. Actual deception of the public or injury to competition need not be shown to constitute a violation. An interesting court case involving these provisions was *Federal Trade Commission v. Pharmtech Research, Inc.* (1983). Based on findings of a National Academy of

Sciences report, the manufacturer of a dietary supplement claimed that consumption of its product—containing vitamins A, C, and E; selenium; beta-carotene; and dehydrated vegetables—would reduce the risk of developing certain cancers. The FTC argued that the company's representations went beyond the report's conclusions and thus were false, misleading, and deceptive. Notwithstanding the conclusions drawn from this prestigious report, an injunction was issued to stop the advertising (Evers, 1988).

U.S. Postal Service

Both civil and criminal fraud statutes are enforced by the USPS. According to Michael Evers, JD (1988), mail fraud statutes are particularly useful for suppression of questionable health care products in view of the United States Supreme Court's consistent rulings that Congress may prohibit any mailing that fosters a scheme that is contrary to public policy *regardless* of its lack of authority to forbid the scheme itself. Federal courts have also held that no proof of actual fraud is necessary in a mail fraud prosecution. Nor is it necessary to show that the victim was misled or that the victim suffered economic loss or damage.

U.S. Department of Justice

Historically, the DOJ has used several criminal statutes usually applied to other criminal offenses for the prosecution of unorthodox medical treatments. Wire fraud, smuggling, and conspiracy statutes have all been routinely used to curtail promotion of unorthodox treatments, especially those used for cancer (Evers, 1988).

In addition to their separate efforts at enforcement, in 1964 the FDA, FTC, and USPS combined with the AMA, American Cancer Society, American Pharmaceutical Association, Council of Better Business Bureaus, and Arthritis Foundation to form the Coordinating Council on Health Information (CCHI). The leader of the council was also the head of the AMA's Department of Investigation. The stated goal of the CCHI was the protection of the public by gathering and disseminating all information involving health quackery (read alternative practices) to its members and particularly law enforcement agencies.

FEDERAL ENFORCEMENT BASED ON LEGAL THEORIES

Constitutional issues, individual rights, and government protection often emerge and clash for consumers and practitioners of alternative medicine. Perhaps one of the most volatile arenas for legal skirmishes involves access to alternative cancer treatments (Evers, 1988). The failure to cure cancer despite the infusion of billions of dollars over decades remains a sore spot for many cancer victims and their survivors. Longer survival rates in some cancers may result from earlier detection using superior technology rather than from any real progress in treatment or cure. Bailar and Smith (1986) note that the selection of one's indicator of cancer survival is crucial to the conclusions drawn. From an epidemiological and statistical standpoint, they find the best measure of progress against cancer is age-adjusted mortality rates. Using these rates, they conclude that

> 35 years of intense effort focused largely on improving treatment must be judged a qualified failure. . . . According to this measure, we are losing the war against cancer. . . . A shift in research emphasis, from research on treatment to research on prevention, seems necessary if substantial progress against cancer is to be forthcoming (pp. 1226, 1231).

Cairns (1985), approaching the cancer question from a clinical and biological standpoint, came to similar conclusions. This frustration has led to a proliferation of alternative treatment modalities, some promising, others useless. And along with that proliferation there have been scores of court cases based on constitutional issues and legal theories.

In a report commissioned by the Office of Technology Assessment, Evers (1988) examined legal constraints on the availability of unorthodox cancer treatments. He notes that federal and state laws and regulations, Medicare and other reimbursement programs, medical practices acts, and malpractice litigation severely limit innovative approaches to cancer cures. Federal courts have considered the legal question of whether the government should be allowed to compel people to choose one system of treatment over another that the individual may prefer, regardless of the basis for that preference.

The constitutional right of privacy and self-determination can be traced back to Supreme Court Justice Cardozo, who in *Schloendorff v. Society of New York Hospital* (1914) stated that "every human being of adult years and sound mind has a right to determine what shall be done with his own body." In 1965 a constitutional right of privacy was established, primarily based on the Ninth Amendment but including also the First, Third, Fourth, and Fifth amendments, guarantees in the Bill of Rights. Confusion still exists in the courts because the Constitution does not explicitly state this right to privacy but finds it under the "penumbras" of various amendments. Those who contend that there is a fundamental right to access to unorthodox cancer treatments do so under the theory that a fundamental right to maintain control over one's body was established under the abortion decisions (Christensen, 1981).

COMPLEMENTING: SEPARATE BUT EQUAL

Can alternative medicine retain its separate identity and values and achieve professional equality with biomedicine? That is, can it ever be *truly* complementary? In carving up the economic pie, formidable and incumbent political and legal forces are arrayed to prevent such equality from happening. These forces must relinquish some of their power (and their share of the economic pie) for true complementary medicine to emerge. Despite the unlikely prospects of that, some promising signs are emerging, more on the individual state level than on the federal level. Examples of this movement will be highlighted in chapter 4, on the power of the state. As is usually the case, economic issues drive political machinery.

Conventional medicine is a $1 trillion a year business. Those with the most to lose tend to bring enormous financial support to bear on protecting their interests. The lure of the developing market, though, makes the battle worth fighting for alternative practitioners.

One way for complementary medicine to emerge in equality is through the blurring of lines between biomedicine and alternative practices. Genuine philosophical differences exist among alternative practitioners over the degree to which they will bend—some say sell out—to be complementary. Licensing of their professions is a two-edged sword (see chapter 4). Although the validation and respectability state licensing brings is most welcome, it is not without its costs. In many cases it requires an alliance in which primary care physicians act as gatekeepers by writing prescriptions for alternatives. Crossover physicians often blur the lines when they practice alternative treatments such as acupuncture and homeopathy, as seen in chapter 7.

AN UNCERTAIN FUTURE

Political and legal forces act either singly or in concert on a national level to limit consumer access to alternative medicine for a variety of reasons. Federal laws and regulations, designed to protect consumers from harm, purportedly for their own good, are often interpreted to protect them from choice as well. Federal health reimbursement programs distribute their limited economic resources almost entirely to conventional biomedical procedures, labeling anything outside mainstream medicine as "experimental." The inroads made by alternative medicine in the creation of a new federal agency is overshadowed by the OAM's relative insignificance in the whole governmental health organization. Although the OAM budget rose from $2 million in 1992 to $7.4 million in 1996, it still represents only 1/5000 of the total NIH budget (Chowka, 1994).

Some prominent political and legal questions remain and are noted below.

OAM—Breaking New Ground or Business as Usual?

Although generally happy with the media exposure, high visibility, and official legitimation that OAM brings to alternative medicine, some proponents have expressed disappointment at its direction. What could have been a ground-breaking opportunity for alternative medicine practitioners to gain official respectability for their professions while maintaining their ideological integrity has not materialized. Instead, there appears to be an effort by the OAM to entice biomedicine into leadership in the agency by invitations to participate in key roles and bestow their approval to alternatives.

In a recent bulletin (AM advisory council, 1995, p. 7), the OAM notes that "rigorous evaluation of the scientific literature will take place to ensure high quality results that are more likely to be accepted as valid by the biomedical community." Similarly, a conference sponsored by the OAM in December 1995, titled "Integration of Behavioral and Relaxation Approaches into the Treatment of Chronic Pain and Insomnia" had an "independent panel, comprised of doctors, nurses, epidemiologists, and statisticians, [who] presented their recommendations . . . at the conclusion of a 3-day technology assessment conference" (NIH panel, 1995, p. 8). Given the noticeable lack of alternative practitioners on the independent panel, this is not exactly the ground-breaking integration nor the professional equality alternative practitioners were hoping for.

Other examples of the direction taken by OAM are found in its structure and publications. Led by a physician who works at Walter Reed Army Institute of Research, the OAM Advisory Council has 18 members—scientists, practitioners, physicians, and other interested parties—the majority of whom are biomedical. Rather than questioning the assumptions of the biomedical research model and concentrating on the development of a holistic paradigm, the research agenda instead reverts to a biomedical methodology in which alternative practitioners will constantly play serious catch-up. OAM publications support the biomedical research models of controlled laboratory experiments, randomized controlled trials, epidemiological and outcomes research, peer review (sometimes called the greatest single obstacle to innovation), and meta-analysis of scientific (i.e., biomedical) literature. Although the OAM bulletin is titled "Complementary and Alternative Medicine," the focus of the office appears to be primarily on complementary medicine under the direction of biomedical methods and personnel. Of the 10 Specialty Research Centers that have been funded, 9 are large biomedical establishments such as the University of Virginia; Columbia University; Beth Israel Hospital, Boston; University of Maryland;

University of California, Davis; Stanford University; University of Medicine and Dentistry, New Jersey; University of Texas, Houston; and the Minneapolis Medical Research Center. Bastyr University is the only alternative organization funded (OAM funds, 1995, p. 8). Further supporting and validating the integration of the biomedical presence in the OAM, an NIH deputy director announced that NIH was considering changing the name of the OAM to the Office of Complementary and Alternative Medicine (AMPAC meeting, 1966, p. 7).

Political Activism—Naïveté Hurts

As baby boomers age and are covered by Medicare, more demands will be made for alternative treatments. The formidable size of this demographic group will be a factor only if its members coalesce as a political force making specific demands of elected officials. Compared to the powerful Jackson Hole Group (a low-profile think tank founded two decades ago by a physician, along with representatives of health maintenance organizations [HMOs], pharmaceutical companies, the American Hospital Association [AHA], and insurance companies), political savvy and lobbying efforts of alternative medicine pale. The Jackson Hole Group came up with the original blueprint for President Clinton's health care plan, with its reliance on managed care, regional purchasing alliances, and HMOs' cradle-to-grave, cost-effective, and efficient health care delivery systems. Recent experience and data have motivated the media and the public to question both the effectiveness and the efficiency of HMOs (Chowka, 1994).

Although currently supported by a groundswell of public opinion, alternative health organizations have not effectively capitalized on this power. Funding for legislative activities is continually short, and infighting over the power roles is evident. Coalitions formed to organize disparate groups come and go with disturbing frequency. Alternative medicine has sometimes been accused of being politically naive, and as a consequence, its lobbying efforts in the past have not been particularly successful. With consumers now solidly and vocally behind alternative medicine, that situation may be changing. The strength of alternative health lobbies is nowhere near that of the AMA, AHA, the pharmaceutical industry, insurance carriers, or other biomedical lobbies, but there are nonetheless attempts to organize consumers under a variety of rubrics—individual freedom, right to medical treatments of their choice, right of privacy, access to "nutriceuticals," and the like.

Alternative health lobbyists do not represent a single, focused force. Rather, there are four distinct lobbying entities representing different interests: (1) practitioners; (2) trade groups; (3) centers, foundations, and institutes; and (4) consumer support and advocacy groups. Coalitions incorporating or representing all four are rare.

Federal Laws and the Health Care Marketplace: Regulation
around the Corner or No End in Sight?

The FDA supported the NLEA because it gave them great regulatory authority to enforce prohibitions against the sale of vitamins and supplements. A groundswell of public opinion led to the repeal of the NLEA and the substitution of the harmless DSHEA. Consequently, the FDA suffered a major slap from the hand of alternative medicine when their enforcement efforts to curtail the marketing of nutriceuticals were halted. At this point the marketing expansion of supplements is escalating rapidly, with inroads into convenience stores, mainstream drug and grocery stores, and other easily accessible markets. It seems unlikely that there will be any further attempts at federal intervention directed to supplements. More interesting, perhaps, is the underground market of FDA-unapproved botanicals, most of which are promoted as cancer cures. These are readily available, often from offshore or border countries.

The Access to Medical Treatments Act (H.R. 2019) is still being debated in Congress. Passage of this bill would grant citizens the right to be treated by health care practitioners with any medical treatment they desire. However, it limits access to those practitioners who have been licensed or certified by a recognized medical or state board. Hence, state licensure carries an incredibly powerful financial incentive, perhaps enough of an incentive to seduce alternative practitioners into compromising their professional ideologies. Even when practitioners are licensed medical doctors, though, access to medical treatments may be denied by government agencies.

Recently, the FDA was accused in Senate hearings of "playing God" with a young boy with brain cancer by first permitting and then arbitrarily denying him access to the synthetic compound antineoplaston. He was deemed by the FDA as no longer being an appropriate subject for the research trials despite the fact that his condition improved with its use. His parents asked a Senate committee debating the Access to Medical Treatments Act, "How many stories do you need to hear? Do you understand that our son is only one example of scores who are being belittled and beat up by a system that only wants familiar [treatments]?" The boy's father disclosed that he continued to get the drug illegally even after FDA disapproval. He told the committee, "The reason I'm willing to tell you that is because that's the kind of thing we shouldn't have to do. Because we have a medicine that's saving our son, our only choice is, do we break the law or let him die? That's sick." The FDA continues to oppose the bill, saying it would be too difficult to ensure that desperate parents are not victimized by fraud (Barker, 1996).

FEDERAL HEALTH CARE REFORM—OPPORTUNITY OR DEATH KNELL?

Politics have laid aside President Clinton's health care plan for now, but calls for reform will surely resurface in the near future regardless of who is in the Oval Office. Most of the plans to date have involved the federal government even more intimately in the nation's health care delivery system than the current system does. Before Medicare was enacted in 1964, health costs had been skyrocketing. Now the nations's total annual health care bill is approaching $1 trillion—14% of the Gross National Product—with no relief in sight. The goal of reform may be more to manage costs than to deliver care.

Many supporters of alternative health care recoil at the direction proposed plans have taken. Reform plans have either ignored the existence of alternatives or considered them "fringe" medicine. Consequently, alternatives proponents to date play no role in the reform of the system. Decisions about medical options would be delegated to regional purchasing alliances and HMOs, possibly creating new cartels in the lucrative conventional medicine area and empowering bureaucrats to a much greater degree. Indeed, more pessimistic critics are of the opinion that national health care reform could well be the end of alternative medicine.

Through HMOs, primary care physicians will act as gatekeepers for their patients. Because peer review by biomedical standards will decide which interventions are acceptable, only approved procedures, such as surgery for cancer, will be employed. If alternative health care is used, it will be with physicians writing prescriptions for chiropractors, naturopaths, acupuncturists, or other licensed alternative health practitioners. Insurance coverage under these plans will most likely be consolidated into those antagonistic to alternatives. The reaction of insurance companies to the Washington State example of mandatory insurance coverage of alternative therapies is a portent of things to come as the companies lobby on the federal level (chapter 6 discusses this issue in greater detail).

CONCLUSIONS

Dichotomies continue to surface in the tug-of-war between alternative medicine and biomedicine. Can we strike a balance between allowing individuals the right to choice of medical treatments versus the collective responsibility of the government to eliminate fraudulent treatments, protecting the public health without protecting the special privilege of biomedical financial interests, cooperative efforts based on a healing team approach of true equality rather than one based on the supremacy of gatekeepers?

Answering these questions requires the proverbial crystal ball for seeing the future. We must note, however, that even without resorting to crystals the political and legal presence of the alternative health movement continues to grow and, in most instances, prosper from the support of an expanding base of consumers. Baby boomers provide a demographic punch to this grass-roots movement as their aging, attitudes, and affluence combine in asserting control over their lives and bodies. Boomers are no strangers to using political and legal power to knock down established ways of doing things. They will continue to be a force well into the next century, so we can expect the face of medicine as we know it to continue changing. Their exposure to New Age trappings made them more comfortable with alternative medicine from the start, and their exposure to other cultures through a global economy promotes ease in understanding and acceptance of customs (including healing customs) different from their own.

Alternative medicine, given these conditions, will not be fading into the sunset in the near future. The question, then, becomes not one of if but of how and to what extent it will be incorporated into the present system of biomedicine. The big legal and political issues revolve around whether alternative medicine will go the already established route of licensure and regulation of its professions. These routes eventually lead to insurance reimbursement, although they will most likely be available only through prescription from a medical doctor. Or will alternative medicine choose a more difficult but innovative route, demanding equal footing on a team with biomedicine? The political power appears to be there for that approach, but it is largely untapped and requires organization, resolve, and political savvy on the part of alternative medicine advocates. This has not historically been their long suit, but times are changing.

There are undoubtedly calls for celebration of alternative medicine's emergence as a visible presence on the federal horizon. It is difficult to look at the legal and political progress of alternative medicine in the past decade and not be impressed with the advances that have been made. Despite that, the political and legal obstacles mentioned above remain formidable and continue to thwart true equality in the combination of allopathic and alternative treatments known as complementary medicine. The reaction of allopathic medicine to challenges of its predominance has been historically recorded and is predictable. They will offer carrots in some instances and sticks in others, but the bottom line is focused on their being in control. The political and legal direction that alternative medicine takes is open to conjecture. As in many instances of federal intervention regarding citizens' health, there may be something for most providers, but slices of the economic pie will most assuredly continue to be unequal. But it's a pretty tempting pie.

4

The Power of the State

Leonard D. Baer and Charles M. Good, Jr.

Laws are felt only when the individual comes into conflict with them.
—Suzanne Lafollette

If you think alternative health care is practiced only on the fringes of the law, think again. The overwhelming majority of alternative health care is legal in all 50 states, albeit with variations in laws and policies within and among states. Legal variations do cause some providers to choose certain states in which to practice their profession. At issue in this chapter: how does the power of the state affect the location and mobility of alternative providers?

Because state laws and policies influence the distribution of alternative care, policymakers must gain a better understanding of what improves or weakens accessibility, availability, and utilization. However, little systematic research exists in any field on alternative health care in the United States, even less on the laws or their impact on providers.

This topic cuts to the heart of the ongoing debate over health reform throughout this country. Every state faces a plethora of unresolved issues of access, cost, and quality of medical care, and debates over health care reform largely exclude the documented utilization of alternative health care. States have the power to severely hamper entire professions, intentionally or unintentionally, not only through straightforward restrictions but also by creating webs of bureaucracy that can decrease access to care.

LEGITIMATION FOR ALTERNATIVE
HEALTH CARE: A TWO-EDGED SWORD

Legitimation encompasses a broad range of factors, most notably stature, acceptance, and professionalization equivalent to biomedicine. Laws and policies play a key role in this and have both a direct and an indirect impact on the legitimation of alternative providers. The public will obviously be wary of any therapy that is banned or deemed fraudulent by the state. At the same time, any state's efforts to revamp health care can have unintended consequences on alternative health practices, such as possible exclusion from health plans and diminished stature as professional health providers.

Some alternative providers fear that the process of legitimation spins a dangerous web not worth the entanglement. State governments would potentially have increased ability to interfere with alternative health practices through regulation. Furthermore, by means of testing requirements or Certificate of Need reviews, a state government could streamline alternative health care toward its conception of acceptable therapies; that is, a health practice with diverse therapies could become altered into a monolithic creation of government or into an indirect creation of biomedicine. Still other alternative providers contend that it is difficult enough to compete with modern medical or biomedical providers; increased competition from other alternative providers would threaten existing alternative practices.

Competition is also a factor for many biomedical providers opposed to legitimation, but it is by no means their only concern. For many biomedical providers, the state's seal of approval on alternative care, regardless of opportunities for legal wrangling, would promote improper health care and would prevent patients from getting medically necessary treatments. They believe legitimation through state control, in heightening the stature of alternative providers, would contradict years of medical training for MDs and other biomedical professionals.

The heightened stature of alternative health care can be demonstrated by the recent creation of the Office of Alternative Medicine at the National Institutes of Health (NIH). NIH has already provided funding for a broad range of projects on therapies such as biofeedback for diabetes, hypnotic imagery for breast cancer, acupuncture and herbal treatment for cancer, acupuncture for osteoarthritis, massage therapy for HIV-exposed infants, and homeopathy for brain injury (NIH, 1997). On the one hand, critics who claim that alternative health care has no scientific validity could only bolster their arguments whenever NIH cannot substantiate claims of efficacy. On the other hand, such critics may need a new line of argument if NIH-funded projects show the validity of numerous alternative therapies. In the future, documented efficacy would make state governments more likely to champion certain applications of alternative care, such as chiropractic for back and neck pain or acupuncture for detoxification from drug dependence.

ALTERNATIVE HEALTH PRACTICES

In any country, the coexistence of alternative health care with biomedicine, home remedies, and self-care reflects multiple views of health care among the general public. In the United States, utilization of multiple health practices has emerged repeatedly in different constructs because of the shifting status of each profession's legitimation and relative power. State laws and regulations also reveal a mixture of therapies and legal approaches that have a direct and indirect influence on legitimation (Table 4.1).

Hypothetically, a newly introduced form of alternative health care may eventually evolve from obscurity to outlaw status to full legal complementarity with biomedicine. The latter achievement is rare, however. Conversely, some forms of care may diminish in stature. Each alternative practice currently stands at a specific level of legal and public acceptance, between the extremes of prohibition and legitimation. The path toward (or away from) legitimation is modeled by Baer (1994a, 1994b; see Fig. 4.1) and demonstrated by the following examples of acupuncture, chiropractic, and homeopathy.

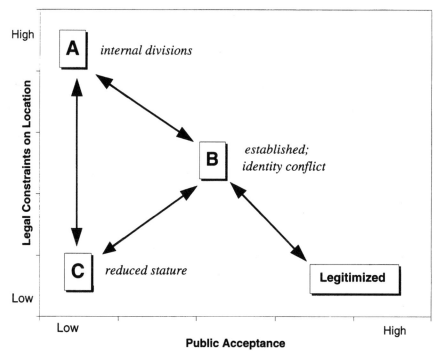

FIGURE 4.1   Model of progression of alternative health providers.

TABLE 4.1 Provider Practice Acts, 1995

State	Acupuncture	Chiropractic	Homeopathy	Naturopathy	Massage
Alabama		✓			
Alaska	✓	✓		✓	
Arizona		✓	✓	✓	
Arkansas		✓			✓
California	✓	✓			
Colorado	✓	✓			
Connecticut		✓	✓	✓	✓
Delaware		✓			✓
District of Columbia	✓	✓		✓	
Florida	✓	✓		a	✓
Georgia		✓			
Hawaii	✓	✓		✓	✓
Idaho		✓			
Illinois		✓			
Indiana		✓			
Iowa	✓	✓			✓
Kansas		✓			
Kentucky		✓			
Louisiana	✓	✓			✓
Maine	✓	✓		b	✓
Maryland	✓	✓			
Massachusetts	✓	✓			
Michigan		✓			✓
Minnesota		✓			
Mississippi		✓			
Missouri		✓			
Montana	✓	✓		✓	
Nebraska		✓			✓
Nevada	✓	✓	✓		
New Hampshire		✓		✓	✓
New Jersey	✓	✓			
New Mexico	✓	✓			✓
New York	✓	✓			✓
North Carolina	✓	✓			
North Dakota		✓			✓
Ohio		✓			✓
Oklahoma		✓			
Oregon	✓	✓		✓	✓

TABLE 4.1 *Continued*

State	Acupuncture	Chiropractic	Homeopathy	Naturopathy	Massage
Pennsylvania	✓	✓			
Rhode Island	✓	✓			✓
South Carolina	✓	✓			
South Dakota		✓			
Tennessee		✓			
Texas	✓	✓			✓
Utah	✓	✓		*a*	✓
Vermont	✓	✓		*b*	
Virginia	✓	✓			
Washington	✓	✓		✓	✓
West Virginia		✓			
Wisconsin	✓	✓			
Wyoming		✓			

Sources: Sale (1995), Mitchell (1995).
a Florida and Utah had practice acts but did not grant new licenses to naturopaths.
b Maine and Vermont have added practice acts for naturopathy.
Note: Some of the states permitting non-MD acupuncture or requiring training for MD acupuncturists did so despite the absence of a practice act. Absence of a practice act does not necessarily mean that a practice is illegal.

Acupuncture, chiropractic, homeopathy, and other alternative health practices exemplify the usefulness and applicability of the model shown in Figure 4.1. The X-axis represents public acceptance of alternative health care, drawing upon Eisenberg et al. (1993). The Y-axis represents the geographical component focusing on the impact of state laws and policies on the locational behavior of alternative health providers. The model provides a context and structure for understanding and predicting the legitimation of alternative health practices.

In Level A professions, such as acupuncture, state laws and policies have a strong bearing on the locational behavior of alternative providers in search of legal status. Chiropractic is in Level B and currently stands as the main alternative competitor to biomedicine. From Level B, a profession can move in one of three directions: (1) decline in popularity and legal acceptance (to Level A), (2) reduced stature and fewer legal constraints (to Level C), or (3) increased stature as a parallel system to biomedicine (to "Legitimized"), which may entail an odd fusion of two health systems (osteopathy, once considered an alternative health profession, became legitimized when its members were accepted into the AMA). In Level C, the power of the state influences locational preferences only in rare cases, such as the recent prohibition of homeopathy in North Carolina. New or little-known forms of alternative health care that do not have any relevant statutes also may be found in Level C.

ACUPUNCTURE

Acupuncture involves the insertion of needles at precise acupuncture points along the body. Acupuncture originated in China thousands of years ago but did not arrive in the United States until around the mid 1800s, when Chinese immigrants found work here building railroads and mining gold. Until the 1970s, after President Nixon's visit to China, the use of acupuncture rarely spread beyond Asian communities in this country (Beinfield & Korngold, 1991). According to a study published in the *New England Journal of Medicine*, it was estimated that less than 1% of the United States population used acupuncture in 1990 (Eisenberg et al., 1993).

Ask acupuncturists about the many styles of acupuncture and, most likely, they will disagree on definitions and classification headings. A sampling of acupuncture styles includes but is not limited to traditional Chinese medicine, five elements, Japanese, medical, auricular/detoxification, French energetic, and Korean hand acupuncture. Many acupuncturists practice herbology in conjunction with traditional Chinese medicine or other acupuncture styles or may combine acupuncture with a broad array of other therapies. For example, many non-MDs extend their practice beyond acupuncture by adding therapies from other health systems, such as zero balancing, craniosacral therapy, nutrition, energy medicine, and massage. Most MD acupuncturists practice medical acupuncture in conjunction with existing biomedical practices. In short, no single acupuncture style has a monopoly on credibility, and many acupuncturists practice multiple styles and combine health systems (Baer, 1994a).

The profession has two competing groups of practitioners in the United States: those who are medical doctors or osteopaths (referred to here as MD acupuncturists) and those who are not (non-MDs). MD and non-MD acupuncturists conflict with each other over perceived competition, differences in approaches to health care, and dissimilar state laws and policies. The latter issue, particularly regarding education requirements, has caused significant tension and rifts among practitioners.

MD acupuncturists express concern that high school graduates, who subsequently receive 2 or 3 years of professional training in acupuncture, demand professional parity with MDs. Even some non-MDs agree that a knowledge of biomedicine can benefit the practitioner's level of competence. Non-MD acupuncturists counter that many MDs lack sufficient training in acupuncture. Two or 3 years of training for non-MDs contrasts with approximately 6 months of training for MDs who join the American

Academy of Medical Acupuncture (AAMA), the major professional association for MD acupuncturists (McDaniels, 1991).

Even this 6-month educational threshold might be too stringent for some
MD acupuncturists: as reported in a popular journal, only about 500 of an
estimated 3000 MD acupuncturists belong to the AAMA ("Alternative
Medicine," 1994). Only about 2,000 of an estimated 6,000–7,000 non-MD
acupuncturists belong to the National Commission for the Certification of
Acupuncture (NCCA, 1993), the major professional association for non-
MD acupuncturists, which has its own set of criteria for membership
(Mitchell, 1995). Because of a lack of licensing for many practitioners in the
United States, the NCCA and AAMA add needed credibility to their respec-
tive members.

In addition to outright restrictions, states have developed several
approaches to regulating non-MD practice, such as required referrals from
biomedical doctors and biomedical supervision, which often limits the
acupuncturist's role to that of a physician's assistant. Applicants wishing to
become licensed or registered acupuncturists (LAc or RAc) usually face
requirements comparable to the NCCA's standards (i.e., educational and
testing requirements). Scopes of practice also can vary sometimes for use of
herbs, nutrition, or precise therapies. Generally, states license, register, or certify non-MD acupuncturists, but these terms are often (but not always) inter-
changeable; one term should not be weighed more favorably than another.

According to the Fetzer Institute's 1995 publication, *Overview of Legislative
Developments concerning Alternative Health Care in the United States* (Sale,
1995), 26 states and the District of Columbia have acupuncture practice acts
for licensure (or the equivalent) of providers. In actuality, sources differ over
the number of states allowing non-MD acupuncture. The difficulty in obtaining a consistent count can be explained by the lack of uniformity in acupuncture laws from state to state, contrasts in the enforcement of restrictive
laws, and recent and ongoing changes in state laws and policies toward
non-MD acupuncture.

As shown in Figure 4.2, most of the states along the Atlantic and Pacific
coasts have acupuncture practice acts, whereas most of the interior states
do not. In examining this coastal pattern, it is interesting that acupuncture
practice acts were first passed in the 1970s in Oregon, Nevada, Hawaii,
California, and, for the most part, other western states. Especially in some
of the states that passed the earliest laws, acupuncture took root in communities with high concentrations of immigrants from China and surrounding
countries. Differences in health-seeking behavior, as well as variations in
cross-cultural acceptance, may partially explain the coastal pattern. Economics, education, and organizational strength also may help explain the
geographical differences. In some states acupuncture practice acts were

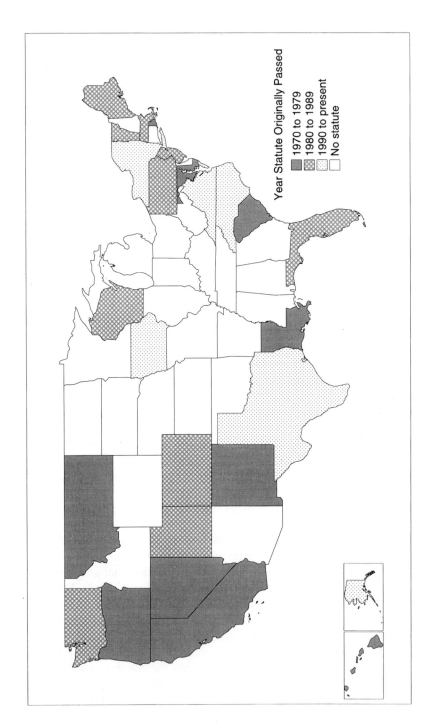

FIGURE 4.2 States with acupuncture practice acts. Adapted from Sale (1995), Mitchell (1995).

passed in response to AMA lobbying for stringent state laws and policies toward non-MD practice (McRae, 1982). Acupuncture's recent introduction to the general public comes into play in shaping the distribution of practice acts. As acupuncture becomes better known, interest in its accessibility and utilization may spread further to the interior cluster of states without practice acts. Passage of new laws would follow.

In states that do not have acupuncture practice acts, acupuncture is generally deemed legal only if it is practiced by a licensed health professional, such as a medical or osteopathic doctor, a podiatrist, or a chiropractor. In a majority of states, MD acupuncturists may practice legally regardless of their training in acupuncture (Mitchell, 1995).

State boards of medicine typically issue and oversee regulations (B. Anderson, Special Counsel, AMA, personal correspondence, January 21, 1993). The Fetzer Institute lists only six states with independent acupuncture boards led by non-MDs (Sale, 1995). There are some surprising complexities involved in obtaining an accurate count of independent boards, including contrasting levels of medical control over acupuncture units within or in relation to medical boards, separate boards for alternative modalities, and separate boards geared specifically toward Oriental medicine. In cases of licensure by separate boards, acupuncturists have greater freedom to practice independently of biomedical control. The resulting increase in autonomy enables acupuncturists to promulgate their own regulations and serves as an important component of legitimation.

CHIROPRACTIC

Chiropractic involves the adjustment and manipulation of the spine and paraspinal tissue to correct or reduce spinal misalignments. The misalignments, according to chiropractic theory, can disrupt the transmission of nerve impulses and impair health. According to estimates by Eisenberg et al. (1993), 10% of the United States population used chiropractic in 1990.

All 50 states and the District of Columbia have licensing requirements for chiropractors. As with acupuncture, uniform testing requirements do not exist. Licensure candidates must abide by state laws dictating the specific required sections of the National Board examinations (Federation of Chiropractic Licensing Boards [FCLB], 1995). Some states' laws appear to provide for reciprocal treatment of chiropractors tested elsewhere, a factor that would enable them to relocate more easily. However, no matter how long a chiropractor has been practicing, he or she faces an almost certain prospect of taking supplemental exams in order to relocate to a new state. Renewal fees also vary from state to state, sometimes by several hundred dollars (FCLB, 1995).

Most states require graduation from a fully accredited college. The United States has 16 chiropractic colleges fully accredited with the Council on Chiropractic Education (CCE), including one that is also accredited by the Straight Chiropractic Academic Standards Association (SCASA) (FCLB, 1995). Of the 16 CCE- or SCASA-accredited colleges, 5 are located in the Midwest (2 in Missouri and 1 each in Illinois, Minnesota, and Iowa), 4 in California, and 2 in Texas. South Carolina, Georgia, New York, Oregon, and Connecticut each have a college. Since the summer of 1993 the United States Department of Education no longer recognizes SCASA as an accrediting authority, although a few states still recognize SCASA accreditation (FCLB, 1995).

State laws and policies toward chiropractic do not appear to foster *straight* or *mixer* populations of chiropractors. The terms "straight" and "mixer" never accurately described the entire population of chiropractors, but a clarification of the terms is nevertheless informative. Historically, on one extreme, some chiropractors would "mix" spinal manipulative therapy with medical diagnoses, ancillary therapies, or even naturopathy, acupuncture, and other health care systems. On the other extreme, "straight" chiropractors would regard spinal manipulative therapy as a corrective procedure, in and of itself, for numerous physical ailments (Wardwell, 1988). Such ailments could include infectious diseases, asthma, allergies, obesity, and diabetes. Indeed, in 1895 in Davenport, Iowa, D. D. Palmer performed the first recorded chiropractic manipulation, not for back or neck pain but for hearing loss (Wardwell, 1988).

Today most chiropractors tend not to be extreme straights or mixers but fall somewhere in between. For example, one chiropractor told the first author (Baer) that he identifies largely with straight chiropractic but still uses vitamin therapy and homeopathy in addition to chiropractic for his patients. Meanwhile, the general public tends to have its own view of chiropractic as an adjunctive therapy to be used for back and neck pain.

Most state laws and policies do not limit chiropractic to spinal conditions, although no state permits chiropractors to write prescriptions or perform surgery. From state to state, some variations exist regarding scope of practice in such areas as physiotherapy, nutritional counseling, treatment of extremities, use of x-ray machines, and schoolchildren's examinations. New York State chiropractors are prohibited from treating communicable or infectious diseases, heart ailments, diabetes, and several other conditions (FCLB, 1995). In 43 states and the District of Columbia, chiropractors have "insurance equality," or equal standing with biomedical providers for insurance coverage of patients (FCLB, 1995). The exact status of insurance equality was unknown or not as clear in three other states. The issue of insurance equality may be directly or indirectly linked to the existence of separate chiropractic boards. As with acupuncture, chiropractors are obviously at a disadvantage if boards of medicine, composed mainly of biomedical doctors, promulgate regulations regarding their profession.

Amid efforts to reach full legal complementarity with biomedicine, chiropractic has faced numerous obstacles imposed by the AMA, as evidenced by the *Wilk v. American Medical Association* (1987) decision in favor of chiropractic. A federal judge ruled that the AMA conspired with other biomedical organizations to discredit chiropractic; furthermore, the AMA had prohibited its members from granting referrals to chiropractors or from having any professional association with them (Injunctive Order, 1987). Whereas such anticompetitive actions are no longer legal, they mirrored earlier AMA efforts against other forms of alternative care, such as homeopathy.

HOMEOPATHY

Homeopathy involves taking an infinitesimal dose of a substance that, if taken in a larger dose, would create symptoms similar to those being experienced. The materia medica of homeopathy, its pharmacopeia, consists of pure substances from animal, vegetable, and mineral products. It is estimated that less than 1% of the United States population used homeopathy in 1990 (Eisenberg et al., 1993).

Only Arizona, Connecticut, and Nevada license homeopathy. Arizona and Nevada have independent homeopathy boards, whereas Connecticut licensure falls under the general authority of the Department of Public Health and Addiction Services. In all other states, homeopathy falls within the legal scope of practice of other licensed health providers (Sale, 1995). Despite the profession's decline in the United States since the 1920s, homeopathy still enjoys popularity throughout much of the world, from Buckingham Palace to India and beyond.

As with chiropractic, the history of homeopathy is intermingled with the history of the AMA. In the 1840s homeopathy became the most predominant form of alternative care in the United States (Coulter, 1982). It was no coincidence that the 1840s also saw the early beginnings of the AMA. The AMA staunchly, and successfully, opposed the practice of homeopathy and enhanced the credibility of biomedicine. Then, in 1910, the Carnegie Foundation, in cooperation with the AMA, issued the Flexner Report, which nearly destroyed homeopathy in the United States (see chapter 5). By the mid 1930s the last homeopathic college, the Hahnemann Medical College of Philadelphia, ceased teaching homeopathy (Coulter, 1982).

In a recent case, after a lengthy court battle the Supreme Court of North Carolina ruled that homeopathy is illegal, thus making North Carolina the only state in the country to prohibit homeopathy (*In re George A. Guess,*

1990). *In re Guess* prompted an outcry from supporters of alternative health care. As a result of subsequent lobbying activity, homeopathy was legalized in North Carolina in the summer of 1993 (Garloch, 1993). Later in the same summer, North Carolina legalized non-MD acupuncture as well. The link between the two changes in legal status reflects a loosely coordinated effort, focused on North Carolina. The abrupt turnabout toward legal acceptance of alternative health care in North Carolina symbolizes a growing movement, crossing professional boundaries, that has the strength to change laws.

BEYOND ACUPUNCTURE, CHIROPRACTIC, AND HOMEOPATHY

According to the Fetzer Institute, only two other alternative health professions have provider practice acts in the United States: naturopathy and massage. Numerous other alternative professions have relevant statutes within medical practice acts targeted at other professions. The following discussion draws on the most comprehensive single document available on the subject (Sale, 1995). As noted earlier for acupuncture, sources differ over the number of states allowing particular health practices.

Naturopathy

Naturopathy, which involves natural principles of health, often combines numerous therapies, such as homeopathy, acupuncture, and hydrotherapy. The profession was at its most popular in the mid-19th century but has declined substantially in popularity since then (Baer, 1992). There are three United States colleges offering degrees in naturopathy, all of which are in the West: Bastyr University in Seattle, Washington; National College of Naturopathic Medicine in Portland, Oregon; and Southwest College of Naturopathic Medicine in metropolitan Phoenix, Arizona (Burton Goldberg Group, 1995).

As of 1996, a total of 11 states have naturopathic practice acts: Alaska, Arizona, Connecticut, Hawaii, Montana, New Hampshire, Oregon, Utah, Washington, and two states newly added to the list, Maine and Vermont. Scope of practice varies from state to state, as naturopathy encompasses a vast array of therapies. A few states, such as Montana and Oregon, permit naturopaths with specialty certification to perform minor surgery or deliver babies. Acupuncture, biofeedback, and massage frequently fall within the scope of practice for naturopaths.

Naturopathy is illegal in some states. For example, Tennessee considers the practice of naturopathy a misdemeanor unless engaged in by MDs (who are not trained to practice it). South Carolina considers the practice of naturopathy a criminal offense for any health provider, licensed or unlicensed.

Massage

Massage therapy has practice acts in 20 states, but one third of those states have enacted their practice acts since 1991. Eight states have independent boards regulating massage. In contrast to most other forms of alternative health care, laws and policies concerning massage also can vary at the local level. The municipal and county laws often supersede state laws and sometimes appear to be in response to concerns about the possibility of sexual massage and prostitution.

Throughout the United States, massage often falls within the scope of practice for other health professions, such as medicine, osteopathy, chiropractic, naturopathy, podiatry, acupuncture, and, most frequently, physical therapy. Some massage acts specifically allow chiropractors and osteopaths to perform massage. Some states view the therapeutic purposes of massage as rather general, without specifying any particular range of conditions. Other states limit massage to stress reduction, increasing range of motion, relieving pain, and other conditions.

ALTERNATIVE HEALTH CARE WITHOUT PRACTICE ACTS

Broadly speaking, most forms of alternative health care have legal sanction only if practiced by a licensed health provider or, in some cases, if the provider does not charge for services. Sometimes states will grant legal sanction if a patient signs an informed consent authorization. However, laws and policies may depend on statutes for other professions. A few examples follow, providing a broad overview of some alternative health professions with applicable laws in more than one state.

Acupressure (acupuncture without needles) and shiatsu (literally, "finger pressure" in Japanese) are often considered in legislation as adjunctive therapies for acupuncture and massage. Biofeedback training—teaching a person how to control the nervous system for stress reduction, asthma, or other conditions—has relevant statutes within practice acts for psychologists or, in some states, physical therapists or naturopaths. Herbology (herbal medicine) is often found within the scope of practice for acupuncturists and naturopaths. Because MDs and osteopaths can write prescriptions, they can also legally prescribe herbs. In some states chiropractors also may practice herbology, and a few states allow unlicensed providers as herbologists. Another therapy, spiritual healing, is specifically exempted from licensure requirements in most states. However, Christian Science has sparked controversy and legal disputes in cases involving practitioners who abandoned biomedical care altogether (*Congressional Quarterly*, 1992).

In some cases, scope of practice acts toward other professions can affect aromatherapy, chelation, polarity therapy, *reiki,* and other alternative practices, although such statutes are the exception rather than the rule. State laws throughout the country do not reference many other forms of alternative health care, such as Ayurvedic medicine, iridology, yoga, flower remedies, and craniosacral therapy.

INTRODUCING THE CASE STUDY

From a geographical perspective, we can examine not only laws and policies but also their impact on alternative health professions. By focusing on issues such as location and movement, a study can raise an array of issues that are seemingly unrelated to geography but that have profound policy implications. Baer's (1994a) study[1] did just that and showed that state laws do affect the geography of providers and, by extension, access to care and legitimation. The research question was straightforward: how do state laws and policies influence the location and mobility of alternative health providers?

The jurisdictions in the study area were limited to Maryland, Virginia, North Carolina, and the District of Columbia. These locations were purposely selected because of wide variations in state laws and policies, variations in the number of practitioners per capita, and geographical proximity (for tracing mobility and boundary effects from one area to another).

Within each jurisdiction, Baer (1994a) sampled acupuncturists, chiropractors, and homeopaths. These health practices provided representativeness among the alternative health professions, sufficiently large sample sizes to enable statistical analysis, and a reflection of different levels of legal acceptance in the United States.

In coordinating the study, developing a database of providers turned out to be a major task because, except for chiropractic, the states did not maintain complete rosters. In some cases, such as homeopathy and acupuncture in North Carolina, lists of providers were obtained even though most of the providers broke the law by practicing there. Extensive lists were developed by summarizing incomplete rosters, contacting national and state associations, manually reviewing names in telephone directories, and building on contacts.

---

[1] Study findings in this chapter are based on Baer (1994a), "Alternative Health Care in the 1990s: the Influence of Legal Constraints on the Locational Behavior of Acupuncturists, Chiropractors, and Homeopaths." Baer (1994b) presented "An Overview of the Influence of Legal Constraints on the Locational Behavior of Alternative Health Providers" on this subject at a 1994 conference.

Separate questionnaires were drafted for acupuncturists, chiropractors, and homeopaths, with only minor variations, and pilot-tested on 10 respondents. The pilot survey, which included in-depth discussions, was one of the most important components of the project because of the valuable input of alternative providers in the project's formulation. The final survey was conducted during the summer of 1993, and a review of the findings was completed in 1994 (Baer, 1994a). Key survey questions focused on the impact of state laws and policies on the location and mobility of alternative providers. Response rates for the survey were as follows: (1) acupuncturists, 64.0% (144 total respondents); (2) chiropractors, 65.9% (203 total respondents); and (3) homeopaths, 69.2% (18 total respondents).

THE ACUPUNCTURE STUDY

In all three states in the study area, state laws and policies underwent major changes only months after the surveys were conducted (Table 4.2). Maryland eliminated its supervision law, changed from registration to licensure, and created a separate Board of Acupuncture for non-MDs. Virginia eliminated its outright prohibition and now allows non-MD acupuncture with required referrals. And in North Carolina, where non-MDs defied the law by practicing and even advertising their services, the state reversed its prohibition of non-MD acupuncture and created a separate Board of Acupuncture.

Study findings showed that legal requirements strongly influence the locational behavior of acupuncturists in states with favorable laws and policies toward non-MD practice. To illustrate this point, compare Virginia with Maryland, two neighboring states. MD acupuncturists constituted 96.4% of Virginia respondents versus a surprising 4.5% in Maryland. Maryland had the highest number of acupuncturists per capita in the study area (1:20,287). Maryland acupuncturists overwhelmingly viewed the legal climate as being especially tolerant. In particular, non-MD acupuncturists in Maryland cited the avoidance of legal prohibition and the simple ability to practice acupuncture at all as influences that affected their decisions to practice in the state.

By contrast, in Virginia non-MD practice was absolutely prohibited at the time of the study. Few respondents there cited the state as having especially favorable laws or policies toward acupuncture. In choosing practice sites, Virginia acupuncturists were mainly influenced by the location of their existing practices in biomedicine. Acupuncture laws tended to be an afterthought, rather than a decisive factor, to geographical decisions for MD acupuncturists. Consistent with this reasoning, over half of all Virginia acupuncturists devoted 10% or less of their practices to acupuncture. By

TABLE 4.2   Major Legal Changes in the Study Area since Summer 1993

Procedure	Legal Change	Maryland	Virginia	North Carolina
Acupuncture	Non-MD acupuncture no longer outlawed	N/A	✓	✓
	Independent acupuncture board established	✓		✓
	Referral requirements established for non-MD acupuncture		✓	
	Referral/supervision requirements removed for non-MD acupuncture	✓		N/A
	Reduction in training for MD acupuncturists[a]	✓		N/A
Homeopathy	Homeopathy no longer outlawed[b]	N/A	N/A	✓

[a] Maryland now requires 200 hours of training for MD acupuncturists, the same as Virginia. North Carolina has no training requirements for MD acupuncturists.
[b] This change in laws took place during the summer of 1993, only hours before the first survey mailing.
Sources: Mitchell (1995), Sale (1995).

contrast, in Maryland, over 60% of acupuncturists devoted 90% or more of their practices to acupuncture.

Virginia and Maryland also contrasted with one another over gender differences. Twenty-five respondents (89.3%) in Virginia were male, compared with only 24 male respondents (36.4%) in Maryland. One explanation: men still dominate many health care professions, as is the case with biomedical doctors and chiropractors. The gender differences therefore can be linked to contrasts between MD and non-MD acupuncture states.

It is more difficult to draw inferences from the unique case of North Carolina, in which 27 of 51 practitioners were non-MD acupuncturists despite prohibitive laws and policies. The non-MDs' open defiance of the law shows that the power of the state cannot always determine health care practice. Nonetheless, it would be foolish to argue that the state does not have a major influence on health care practice and legitimation. All states in the study area do indeed show at least some relation between legal tolerance and choice of a practice site.

A non-MD respondent in Maryland offered an insightful comment that aids in understanding the relation between legal tolerance and locational behavior:

> The "location" of a practice is not always the location of the established office. "Have needles will travel" is the theme of many practitioners who feel free to treat in states other than their home office state. Thus, the laws may

have an influence on where the home office is located but may have little/no bearing on the freedom one feels to treat in non-licensed states.

Non-MDs face legal barriers, even in more tolerant states. Some acupuncturists expressed concerns about the ability to join managed care plans or, once included, the ability to receive payment. Also, a number of non-MD respondents complained about Maryland's supervision law, which required acupuncture patients to have a prior, biomedical examination and referral. "It undermines the public's confidence in an acupuncturist's ability and heightens the stature of doctors," a Maryland non-MD acupuncturist commented on the survey. Non-MDs expressed concerns about delays in treatment and limitations on the patient's access to care. Few respondents mentioned the supervision law as a factor influencing locational preference.

Instead, practitioners in all states frequently mentioned legality, ability of non-MDs or MDs to practice, and concerns about licensure. With Virginia's acupuncture laws changing to allow non-MD acupuncture, some practitioners from neighboring states expressed strong interest in practicing there. For example, a non-MD acupuncturist, who commuted from Virginia to Maryland, said that when the law changes, "I'm going to give the neurologist [who practices acupuncture] a run for his money." "I'd love to be able to practice acupuncture in Virginia when the law changes," another Maryland acupuncturist commented.

The influx of practitioners causes reasonable alarm for some MD acupuncturists, concerned about quality of care and competition. Many acupuncturists in Virginia object to the legal change. An osteopathic physician wrote on the survey: "I am concerned about upcoming changes in the VA laws which will allow nonphysicians to practice acupuncture. Specifically, the nonphysicians lobbyist groups have tried to restrict physicians' practice of acupuncture. This arrogance could adversely affect patients under their care." A Virginia MD explained his concerns this way: "Acupuncture is a medical modality of treatment, as is surgery, medications, and physical therapy, respiratory therapy. It is not a complete independent system. It is part of and belongs in the medical treatment modalities."

The pattern of conflicts within the field of acupuncture fosters state laws and policies that favor or disfavor MDs or non-MDs. In turn, the legal constraints lead to deepening rifts within the profession.

THE CHIROPRACTIC STUDY

Study findings indicate that most chiropractors view chiropractic as a full health profession in its own right, at least parallel to biomedicine. Approximately 75% or more of chiropractors in Maryland, Virginia, and North Carolina responded, respectively, that chiropractic should be used, for "strengthening immunity," "neonatal care," and "prenatal care." The survey did not include a definition for chiropractic, so some providers may have answered for ancillary therapies, such as physiotherapy or nutritional counseling, in addition to spinal manipulative therapy.

The contradictory perceptions of many patients and chiropractors about the breadth of the profession can constrain locational preference. In fact, roughly half of all chiropractors in the study area have practiced their entire careers for the same number of years "in total" as "in this county" (10 to 12 years on average, depending on the state). The relationship between many chiropractors and new patients continues to be somewhat clouded by divergent views about the breadth of chiropractic. As a result, a number of chiropractors will be less likely to move away from existing practices to locations with relatively uncertain patient bases. Time and money spent building a practice and winning new adherents might be wasted by relocating to another county or state and starting a practice anew.

Numerous legal, social, and economic factors also help explain the limited mobility of chiropractors. State laws and policies, such as insurance equality, testing requirements, scope of practice, and reciprocity, have impeded the mobility of at least half of all chiropractors in the study area. Among respondents who reported some legal impedance, most cited only a minor impact of legal constraints on mobility. Chiropractors also may stay in the same location because of strong community ties. Moreover, the financial costs of opening new practices serves as a strong incentive to remain in the same location.

Other study findings reveal a moderate but unclear relation between the locational preferences of chiropractors and legal constraints. For example, in 1993, Maryland had the lowest number of chiropractors per capita (1:10,216) of any state in the entire country.[2] At the same time, chiropractors there reported that the state had a favorable legal atmosphere. By comparison, in North Carolina, chiropractors reported approximately the same degree of legal tolerance as in Maryland, despite having a much larger number of chiropractors per capita (1:6,499). A key distinction helps clarify why Maryland and North Carolina share common ground in having favorable legal perceptions: Maryland and North Carolina have separate chiropractic boards; Virginia does not. It is no small coincidence that legal constraints disproportionately influence the choice of practice site for chiropractors in Maryland and North Carolina.

---

[2] The FCLB (1993) data are based on the total number of chiropractors licensed in a state, as opposed to the total number actually practicing in a state. The latter would include even fewer chiropractors per capita.

Scope of practice, reciprocity, and insurance opportunities affect not only locational decisions but also practices in general. Regarding insurance, chiropractors do not face the same degree of exclusion from managed care plans as do other alternative providers, no doubt because chiropractors are frequently viewed as specialists for back and neck pain. Nonetheless, on the survey, chiropractors frequently wrote special comments about the importance of insurance equality and financial considerations for their practices.

One Virginia chiropractor explained that, in focusing on laws and not on economic concerns, the survey "missed the point" of why people choose certain practice locations:

> What a person is looking for is that part or small area of the city or county they are going to practice in that has the highest per capita income, the largest *stable*, not transient, population (regardless of their income level) and the greatest longevity (of the population) at their jobs. These people have two things: disposable income (because chiropractic isn't covered by all insurances) and generally a better quality insurance than a transient population would have.

A Maryland chiropractor commented on the impact of insurance coverage on access to chiropractic: "We have to turn a great number of patients away because their health insurance (especially HMOs and corporate-based plans) does not include chiropractic coverage." A chiropractor in North Carolina made the following comments about the problems inherent in insurance coverage for chiropractic care:

> In my location it is very difficult to obtain access to HMOs and PPOs. I have been told "we have a chiropractor we refer to" but no name is given when requested. My patients who belong to these plans have difficulty obtaining chiropractic care; most of them pay cash to see me. Why cash? Because they are refused referral to a chiropractor by their health plan's doctor.

The MDs who are responsible for making such referrals tend to have limited conceptions about chiropractic, and chiropractors also disagree among themselves about the scope of the profession. Through a better understanding of chiropractic and its geographical characteristics, researchers can better understand the profession's uncertain status as a limited health care profession, as well as the financial and competitive constraints involved in building a patient base. This section therefore serves as an exploratory underpinning for future research.

THE HOMEOPATHY STUDY

Survey results for homeopathy are drawn from a small population, and do not necessarily have any statistical validity. The findings are indicative of homeopathy in general and come at a time when many advocates of homeopathy claim a resurgence of the profession in this country.

Legal efforts aside, acupuncture and chiropractic can both be measured easily in terms of the number of practitioners per capita. In homeopathy, though, a 1993 count of practitioners totaled only 5 in North Carolina, 10 in Virginia, 10 in Maryland, and 3 in the District of Columbia. The directory of the National Center for Homeopathy (1993) listed approximately 315 professional homeopaths in the entire country. Some researchers have estimated the total number of homeopaths to be over 1,000, perhaps because of lay homeopaths (e.g., Clark, 1993; *Congressional Quarterly*, 1992).

Lay homeopaths, practitioners with no state licensure in a health profession, compensate for a lack of access to professional homeopathic services. Many lay homeopaths limit their practices to family and friends. Others practice without legal sanction, charging for services and building professional practices. Dana Ullman (personal correspondence, March 12, 1993), who writes frequently about homeopathy, estimated that there are several hundred such practitioners in the country.

A professional homeopath remarked to a Virginia study group that many lay homeopaths serve a useful purpose in providing needed access to care. Even the broad array of educational backgrounds among homeopaths does not produce any apparent intraprofessional division, although further study is needed to confirm this finding. The 18 respondents in the homeopathy survey included veterinarians, biomedical doctors, PhDs, dentists, nurses, and a chiropractor. With a near absence of homeopaths in many areas, homeopaths of varied backgrounds often work with each other to provide access to care.

The limited findings here showed certain similarities within the profession: most homeopaths have relocated from their original counties of practice, are in their 40s, and practice classical homeopathy (i.e., each remedy is derived from a single substance). Some practitioners also combine homeopathy with other healing arts.

Although homeopathy no longer poses a competitive threat to biomedicine in the United States, a few respondents commented about problems with the biomedical community. One homeopath confided: "I have a clinic in the lower level of my home, due to need for a low profile so minimum harassment will occur—my colleagues have been severely harassed by AMA."

North Carolina's recent prohibition of health care that does not meet "acceptable and prevailing standards" has led several respondents to consider legal constraints before choosing a state in which to practice. Despite such apprehension, locational preferences of homeopaths are often determined by issues that have, at one time or another, affected anyone's locational preferences: family, hometown, and schools for their children. With a larger population of homeopaths and with the possibility of increased stature as health professionals, future results can be expected to reveal more complex findings.

CONCLUSIONS

The power of the state has an impact on the locational choices of alternative providers to varying degrees, depending on the particular profession and level of legal acceptance. State governments affect the spatial patterns of alternative providers by creating, in many cases, barriers to movement even between neighboring states. Consider licensed non-MD acupuncturists. In some states they cannot legally practice across a neighboring state's border without encountering prohibitive laws and policies. MD acupuncturists also face restrictive legal barriers, such as educational and licensing requirements, that stand in the way of opening new practices. However, general statements about the location and mobility of acupuncturists usually do not hold true for chiropractors, homeopaths, and other providers. Each group and sometimes, subgroup of alternative providers has a distinct geography, in large part because of contrasting levels of legal acceptance, legitimation, demographic variables, and economic considerations.

Non-MD acupuncturists face a strong influence of state laws and policies on locational behavior. MD acupuncturists, on the other hand, tend to practice in the same locations previously used for practicing biomedicine.

Legal constraints do not dramatically affect the locational preferences of chiropractors but nonetheless have a moderate impact on choosing a site at which to practice chiropractic. Chiropractors did express strong concerns over variations in insurance equality and the lack of uniform testing requirements.

North Carolina's recent prohibition of homeopathy has attracted nationwide attention among alternative providers and has impeded practitioners from moving there. With legal status and the absence of laws and policies regulating homeopathy in all but a handful of states, homeopaths generally face few legal restrictions on locational preference.

Despite the power of the state, progress toward legitimation can occur independently of state sanction. Communities view providers with respect or disdain based on views at the local level, not merely the views of policymakers and state legislators (Last, 1990). Nonetheless, the state ultimately plays a decisive role in any alternative health practice's legitimation.

Public legitimation also can be influenced by word of mouth, professional competition, news coverage, individual personalities of providers, bedside manners, and the familiarity of a health care setting. Insurance companies serve as another component of legitimation. They may increase access to care by including alternative care in their health plans. Conversely, they may destroy opportunities for alternative health care by denying or limiting coverage.

Entire health professions or certain applications of a given health care system may be pushed underground because of medical gatekeeping at insurance companies. A North Carolina chiropractor summed up the views of many alternative providers when he commented, "There should not be `medical gatekeepers' directing patients with regard to chiropractic. Not all MDs understand what chiropractic physicians do." Chiropractic's political and financial clout prevents the profession from being forced into an underground phenomenon. The future is less certain for less entrenched forms of alternative care, but a patient's ability and willingness to pay for services will always supersede any insurance restrictions.

Ongoing studies at NIH, focusing on the scientific validity of alternative therapies, will affect the decisions of insurance companies and even of state legislatures regarding the future and scope of alternative health care. If new studies reveal certain alternative care as efficacious, prospects for legitimation and corporatization will certainly be enhanced. The power of the state aside, health professions can grow or wither by their own merit or misfortune.

Recent events depict a pattern of increased legal acceptance for alternative health care (e.g., changes in acupuncture laws in Virginia, Maryland, and North Carolina and changes in homeopathy laws in North Carolina). The changes should be viewed in the context of overall health policy because alternative health care frequently complements biomedicine in health care. However, until now policymakers, public health officials, and academic researchers have largely considered health care the exclusive domain of biomedicine, without examining accessibility and utilization patterns of alternative health care.

Relatively unexplored and crucial issues affecting alternative health services include legal acceptance, legitimation, scope of practice, and the unity or divisiveness within alternative professions. This chapter calls attention to these and other legal and social issues that should be included in statewide and nationwide debates over health reform.

5

Paradigms and Politics: Redux of Homeopathy in American Medicine

Kristen S. Borré and James L. Wilson

When we try to describe experience with classical logic, we put on a set of blinders,
so to speak, which not only restricts our field of vision, but also distorts it.
These blinders are the set of rules known as classical logic. . .
The only problem is that they do not correspond to experience.
—Zukav (Dancing Wu Li Masters)

One hundred years ago, American medicine was characterized by a plurality of health care systems. Prominent among these systems were allopathy, the nascent system of biomedicine familiar to us today, and homeopathy, an equally historic system common in Europe and enjoying a resurgence in the United States. The complex history of the relationship between these two medicines intersects with the history of the American Medical Association and its accreditation policies, the successful growth of large pharmaceutical corporations, and the unwillingness of homeopaths to share their successful treatments with their allopathic colleagues. The two paradigms, or explanatory models, of medical practice contrasted boldly and led to emotional battles among physicians and schools of medicine. It was heresy on the part of either system to give credence to the other. The problem addressed in this chapter is to examine how these two systems of medicine, each owning successes in treatment of different disorders and diseases, became alienated from one another and to explain how homeopathic medicine has recently become a popular form of alternative medical care in the United States. To begin to understand this story, it is important to look at the concept of paradigm in different systems of thought or cultures. From there, homeopathy as a form of medicine and a brief history of its practice are developed. Finally, cultural, historical, and political questions about homeopathy as practiced by MDs and other licensed health providers in the United States are raised for the reader's consideration.

PARADIGM, CULTURE, AND MEDICINE

Cassidy (1994, pp. 6–12) addresses the differences in the paradigms of reductionist or scientific explanatory models such as those used by allopathic physicians in biomedical practice and the holistic or relational explanatory models often used by physicians and healers subscribing to alternative health care practices, such as acupuncture or homeopathy. She offers the metaphor of the "whole ball of string" to help professionals come to grips with the limitations of their own paradigms and to move beyond them, leaving fear of the unknown and defensiveness behind. In the whole-ball-of-string model, each discipline comprises a single strand of reality that can be used to explain a particular phenomenon, but the larger picture of reality can be gained only as all the strings come together through twists and turns and knots to explain a composite of phenomena. The twists and turns and knots allow people of different backgrounds opportunity to work together to unravel the mysteries their separate disciplines cannot solve. The metaphor of the ball of string allows professionals from differing paradigms to focus on the problem at hand and on what each has to offer rather than on the correctness of a single professional paradigm.

The American health care industry has created a health-conscious society with a certain worldview—that health can be improved or restored in the medical marketplace. Physicians are in control of this marketplace, along with insurance companies, the government, and hospitals. For example, residents of a community with high cancer rates saw toxic waste as the source of their cancer. Physicians at the nearby cancer center treated the individual cancer patients as unique cases and identified cancer causation at a personal level (Balshem, 1991). Physicians working within the biomedical, systemic model of cancer were not trained to consider examining and treating the endemic cancer problem as a community problem. The causes of cancer were sought within the patient's own body and mind. If cancer developed, then the patient's own body had failed. The focus was on the patient who, through some personal failing, had acquired cancer and, through heroic efforts to fight the cancer with the physician as coach, could make amends for the prior failing and survive (Balshem, 1991).

Because of its reductionist paradigm biomedicine does not see the patient in a holistic manner as part of the larger community and its environment.

If the patient decides to enlist an alternative health care system that is meaningful in the way he or she conceives the disease process, the biomedical physician considers such a choice dangerous and wasteful of money. The alternative healer also can discourage the patient from getting biomedical help. A standstill between the two healers can catch the patient in the middle, obstructing communication among the healers and the patient.

The model of how to practice medicine, including patient assessment and disease management, is acquired in medical school and residency programs and is carefully monitored by clinical faculty. This biomedical model is supported by the political and economic structure of the health care industry, including pharmacological corporations, insurance companies, and professional medical associations. If Cassidy's whole-ball-of-string approach was adopted by both allopathic and alternative physicians, the patient would be able to focus, with the physicians, on finding the best method for living with the disease or curing it. Exploring prevention of disease and analysis of the role of the community and environment in producing high mortality rates constitutes another string, which could meet the community's need to address its beliefs of causation.

The links between cultural models also are served by the role of the reductionist paradigm and scientific method in biomedicine in explaining disease and treatment in terms of physiology, anatomy, and biochemistry, the "basic sciences" of medicine (Gillett, 1994). Among American families who have lost children to infectious diseases and parents to heart disease, the "miracle drugs"—penicillin, the polio vaccine, cholesterol-lowering medications, and beta-blockers—are success stories that build confidence in allopathic medicine. The bottom line is that no medical paradigm can be widely accepted without having significant successes. Homeopathy provided the successful treatment for cholera and other infectious diseases of the 19th and early 20th centuries. Biomedical miracle drugs were a significant factor that moved the public away from homeopathy.

Today the increased interest in homeopathy may be explained by the lack of success of biomedicine in curing diseases such as AIDS, multiple sclerosis, cancer, asthma, lupus, migraine, and arthritis. Frustrations with these diseases lead the hopeful public to alternative therapies. The alternative paradigm of homeopathy is rooted in Western scientific method but uses scientific theories for explanation different from those of biomedicine. When patients with chronic illnesses fail to find help through biomedicine, they will take advantage of alternative systems to find comfort and cure. This may be one reason that cancer patients are the most frequent users of alternative medicine (Brown, Cassileth, Lewis, & Renner, 1994).

The American public is willing to embrace alternative medicine, with about 33% of the population using alternative therapies (Eisenberg et al.,

1993). The challenge of alternative medicine is whether or not the dominant cultural model in the United States, biomedicine, and the political and economic forces that support it will be open to embracing other models of healing and health maintenance. These phenomena will not require biomedical physicians to admit failure or the frailty of the biomedical model but to demonstrate their willingness to consider other possibly successful approaches to healing and curing. Viewing medicine as a cultural system structured by a specific paradigm assists this shift of meaning in biomedicine. The opportunity exists to expand health care and healing beyond the limits of the concept of any one paradigm using the whole-ball-of-string model (Cassidy, 1994). This metaphor allows us to visualize a humanistic schema in which partnerships can develop among a variety of healers, the patient, and the lay and health care communities to develop new strategies for research, diagnosis, treatment, and health maintenance in diverse populations (Gillett, 1994).

HOMEOPATHIC HEALTH CARE: THE CURRENT STATE

Homeopathic medicine shares with Western biomedicine its history and organization of formal professionalized health care. Scientific research rooted in standard clinical trial methodology supports the efficacy of many remedies (Ullman, 1995). A major question in the study of alternative medicine is why homeopathic medical practice has become relegated to the same category of respect among biomedical physicians as folk traditions such as root doctoring and talking the fire out of burns. Why is it viewed as heresy and "hocus-pocus," as a physician with early training in both homeopathy and allopathy referred to it in a medical school clinical skills course? As late as 1900, 15% of American physicians were practicing homeopaths, graduating from 22 homeopathic medical schools and practicing in over 100 homeopathic hospitals (Ullman, 1991). Throughout the 20th century homeopathy has become professionally discredited and abandoned by the majority of practitioners in spite of demonstrated success in cholera treatment in homeopathic hospitals at the turn of the century (Kaufman, 1971) and in modern clinical trials (Ullman, 1995). Testimonials and writings by public figures like John D. Rockefeller and Louisa May Alcott demonstrate the widespread cultural acceptance of homeopathy in the United States at an earlier time (Ullman, 1991).

The eclipse of homeopathy in American medicine can be partially explained by fundamental differences in the theory of disease and treatment methodology between biomedicine (allopathic) and homeopathic medicine. Biomedicine and homeopathic models are distinct from one another, reflecting divergent worldviews. Biomedical physicians treat illness by focusing on fighting the disease condition with drugs that weaken and destroy the pathogens. In contrast, homeopaths focus on treating disease by using the Law of Similars. This law and related laws of modern homeopathy were developed in the late 18th century by Dr. Samuel Hahnemann, a German physician and writer. The Law of Similars states that medicines that produce the same symptoms in the well person as observed in the sick will cure the disease.

Models of patient care can differ from one another based on the nature of physical examination for diagnosis, the role of the patient in treatment and wellness, and the prescription of medicines. But paradigmatic differences alone cannot account for the degree of animosity felt by biomedical physicians for homeopathy. Historically, there can be found a point of tangency between the practices in Greek philosophy and medicine, early biology, and natural history. Additional explanation of the divergence can be found within the historical context of the political economy of health care and medicine in America. Here, questions of authority and power, control of capital and markets, and medical ethics are embedded in the struggle of homeopathy and biomedicine for cultural, political, and economic hegemony.

HOMEOPATHY AS A PROFESSIONAL HEALTH CARE SYSTEM

Homeopathy[1] is a medical approach that respects the wisdom of the body. It is an approach that utilizes medicines that stimulate the body's own immune and defense systems to initiate the healing process. It is an approach that individualizes medicines according to the totality of the person's physical, emotional, and mental symptoms. It is an approach that is widely recognized as safe (Ullman, 1991, p. 3).

ORIGINS OF HOMEOPATHY

The earliest record of homeopathic medicine dates back to Hippocrates in the 5th century BC. He developed a system of healing based on the principle

---

[1] This differs from the model of complementary medicine presented in chapter 2, which categorizes homeopathy in the alternative body healing quadrant. In this chapter, Borré and Wilson consider homeopathy only as it is practiced by licensed health care providers, which means only a degree from a professional medical, nurse practitioner, physician assistant, naturopathic, or chiropractic school can provide the legal means to practice any form of medicine and then only under the authority of state licensure. In some states homeopaths must be MDs.

that "like cures like." Hippocrates also asserted that disease was the result of naturalistic forces external to the body. He believed that the body had the power to heal itself but that medicinal remedies based on finding the one that could produce symptoms similar to those observed in the patient would enhance the healing process. Hippocrates was the first to attempt scientific proof of an herbal medicinal. He proved that white hellebore (*Veratrum album*) used in very small doses was effective in the treatment of cholera (Lockie & Geddes, 1995, p. 10). Hippocrates argued against the Law of Contraries—that a remedy should be given that produces the opposite symptoms in a healthy person: the medical treatment theory of the day.

Roman physicians from the 1st to 5th centuries developed elaborate pharmacopeias to use in Law of Contraries treatments, and Hippocrates' medical practice became obsolete. The Romans emphasized theories of structure and function of the human body, as exemplified by the work of Galen and others, but did not develop the actual practice of medicine. The Persians and Muslims preserved Roman and Greek knowledge of medicine throughout the European Dark Ages; and in the 16th century, European advances in medicine resumed (Lockie & Geddes, 1995, p. 10). During this period the foundations for modern chemistry were laid, and the Law of Similars was revived but then ignored. The Law of Similars concept reentered medical thinking in 1790, when Samuel Christian Hahnemann demonstrated its efficacy with his first proving of cinchona as a cure for malaria. According to the Law of Similars, this was not because of its astringent properties but its ability to induce consistent malarial symptoms in healthy persons.

Hahnemann, whose background was chemistry and medicine, kept detailed notebooks of his "provings" on other herbal substances used as medicines. He was then able to record levels of significant symptoms associated with each "drug" and to elaborate a "drug picture" for each. From this empirical work he induced the principle of the Law of Similars, a rediscovery that would establish a new system of scientific medicine (Lockie, 1989; Ullman, 1991). The scientific rationale for homeopathy and the basis of Hahnemann's return to the practice of medicine was his book *The Organon*, published in 1810 (Hamlyn, 1979). Apprentices followed his work through the 19th century and continued his method of provings, experimenting with drug dilutions in clinical practice in both Europe and America.

SOCIAL AND POLITICAL CONFLICT WITH HEROIC BIOMEDICINE IN THE UNITED STATES

Reviews of the history of homeopathy in Europe, India, and the United States are found in several scholarly volumes, including Coulter (1975, 1977,

1981), Gevitz (1988), Kaufman (1971), and Ullman (1991). The following review is not meant to be complete but only to sketch how differences in professional paradigms or explanatory models can be politicized in societies in which there is monetary and social power to be gained.

Into the mid-1800s in the United States, biomedicine depended on heroic or drastic practices such as bloodletting and the use of purgatives and emetics to treat patients. Such practices were justified within a medical humors paradigm of human physiology. In most cases treatment by these methods was the last resort and often unsuccessful. George Washington was bled to death after being unable to shake an infectious disease (Ullman, 1991). Hahnemann's followers decried these methods as inhuman and dangerous and offered a more holistic, humanist, personal method of treating illness. In most cases this method was more successful because it subscribed to the axiom that the physician was to "do no harm" in the course of the treatment (Kaufman, 1971).

Homeopathic medical schools began to grow in large numbers, and at one time in the 19th century homeopathic hospitals outnumbered allopathic ones. Homeopaths did not allow allopaths to treat patients in their hospitals, and vice versa. The lines of conflict for control of the developing health care profession were drawn in these ways early on. Biomedical physicians had a difficult time dismissing homeopaths because they were medically trained physicians, unlike folk practitioners such as herbalists (Coulter, 1981). As homeopathy grew in success and popularity with the American public, biomedical physicians' attacks became more public and intensified. Oliver Wendell Holmes led a famous literary attack on homeopathy, and local medical associations began excluding any physician who practiced homeopathy (Kaufman, 1971).

When the American Medical Association (AMA) was formed, it actively denied membership to any physician not trained in allopathic schools or who practiced homeopathy. In 1855 the AMA purged any physician from its ranks who even consulted a homeopathic doctor (Ullman, 1991). One physician was expunged for consulting with his wife about a patient. She, like many women physicians, was a trained homeopath. Another physician was expelled for purchasing lactose from a homeopathic pharmacy (Coulter, 1981). The AMA considered homeopathy immoral, illegitimate, and "unmanly"; opposition was based not on scientific evaluation of its merits but on fear of it as a competitor. Geographically, the AMA was successful in excluding homeopaths in all states but Massachusetts, and it was in Massachusetts that the medical education of homeopaths had the most success.

Homeopaths were often physicians who were denied access to allopathic medical schools because of gender, social class, or lack of money.

Homeopathic schools were less expensive and were open to women (Kaufman, 1971). The first women's medical college was a homeopathic institution, founded in Boston in 1848. In 1873 it merged with Boston University, another homeopathic medical school (Abrams, 1985; Ullman, 1991). Abolitionists, Quakers, and African Americans were also strong supporters of homeopathy. The Protestant clergy openly supported homeopathy as a form of medicine because of its holistic approach and because they were opposed to dependence on addictive drugs, often recommended by biomedical physicians. The difficulties of homeopathy in the South are linked to homeopathy's support by progressives such as abolitionists (Ullman, 1991). This historical context helps explain why North Carolina has been one of the most difficult states for homeopathic physicians to develop practices in.

Medical education was a major front for the conflict. The AMA would not accept the degree of any physician who had a homeopathic physician as instructor, as evidenced by the signatures of instructors required on the diploma for graduation; yet Boston College, Hahnemann Medical College, and the Universities of Iowa, Michigan, and Minnesota were among the medical schools teaching homeopathy (Ullman, 1991). The scientific training of biomedical and homeopathic physicians was identical. Even the *Journal of the American Medical Association* reported that homeopaths scored higher and passed medical boards more frequently than did biomedical physicians ("Medical Education & State Boards of Registration," 1909).

Homeopathy was weakened by several historical events in the early 20th century, well described in Coulter (1981). To summarize them briefly, a combination of political maneuvering by the AMA and the Carnegie Foundation led to a ranking system for medical schools based on allopathic emphasis on the biomedical model and study of pathology (established with the Flexner Report of 1910). This led to the decline of homeopathic colleges, from 23 in 1900 to 2 in 1923 (Kaufman, 1971). John D. Rockefeller was treated solely by homeopaths and instructed his estate to endow homeopathic colleges to assure their survival, but his financial investor gave the money to allopathic colleges instead because of his own affiliations with allopathic medicine. To compete with allopathic colleges, homeopathic colleges had to provide course instruction in pathology and biochemistry that diminished the rigorous approach of homeopathic education that had made the homeopathic colleges so successful.

The AMA eventually dropped its ban on homeopaths, and drug companies began deriving medicines from homeopathic formulations that biomedical physicians administered in large doses. This approach replaced the heroic medical practices of the 19th century and was more successful with the public. As a bonus, biomedical physicians could make more money because they could treat more patients. Finally, a homeopath's charges were much lower than those of allopathic doctors, and they spent as much as 10 times longer in diagnoses and treatment. No one thing, like the singular attacks of the AMA, led to the decline of homeopathy. Instead, historical momentum against homeopathy climaxed through the solidification of economic and political powers of biomedical physicians, their financial backers, the growing drug companies, and the institutionalization of medical school ranking and accreditation using biomedical paradigms (Kaufman, 1971). The conflict between biomedical physicians and homeopaths began with different paradigms of medical practice, guarded jealousies, and uncompromising loyalty to the paradigm that was self-serving for the physicians, often leaving the patient's health care needs unmet. It ended with the formalized incorporation of the biomedical paradigm within the governing, cultural, economic, and political structures of the United States.

MODERN HOMEOPATHY

As a professionalized health care system, modern homeopathic practice is best understood in terms of its (1) theory, (2) formal education, (3) delivery system, (4) pharmaceutical and treatment materials support system, (5) legal and economic regulation, and (6) public expectations on the role of medicine.

THEORY AND RESEARCH

The biomedical theory supporting homeopathy is found in quantum physics and the new physics of Prigogine (Prigogine & Stengers, 1984) and Jantsch (1980). In his medical classic, Cannon (1942) argues that the body is a self-regulating system able to defend and heal itself. Symptoms of illness indicate that the body's defenses are activated to heal itself. Homeopathy works by helping the body heal itself through stimulating or calming the immune system with micro-doses of remedies that cause the symptoms of illness in healthy individuals. Biological structures are known to depend on consistent patterns to adapt to environmental stresses and to maintain stability and resilience. Homeopathic treatment helps the individual human body return to and maintain the natural consistent pattern that results in a state of health for that person.

Three assumptions underlie principles of homeopathic therapy. First, symptoms are signals that the human organism is attempting to respond to a particular stress or infection (Ullman, 1995). Second, multiple symptoms do not indicate multiple diseases: most symptoms of illness share a fundamental cause within the body's immune system. Third, when the physician is able to determine the most significant symptom or complex of symptoms, the underlying cause of the illness can be determined and treated with small doses of the appropriate remedy.

Three empirically established laws of homeopathic practice are supported by these assumptions. First, the previously discussed Law of Similars is homeopathy's central principle. Second, the Law of Individuation, shared with biomedical physicians, states that each individual is unique, requiring independent observation, diagnosis, and treatment within all domains of his or her being, including physical, mental, social, and spiritual aspects (Lockie, 1989). Third, the Law of Minimal Doses underlies the preparation of all homeopathic remedies and is the most controversial in relation to biomedical practice.

Homeopathic remedies are based on mineral, herbal, and animal substances known to produce certain consistent symptoms in organisms. Each substance is diluted with distilled water or ethyl alcohol and vigorously shaken. Serial dilutions increase the potency of the remedy (Ullman, 1995). Serial dilutions of very potent or strong remedies can be produced in which no molecules of the original medicinal substance remain. Biomedical physicians, using theory based on chemistry, pharmacology, and disease within the paradigm of the medical model, consider such remedies ineffective. Homeopaths argue that the resonance, energy, and pattern of the original substance have physically altered the water solution and that the physics of that pattern, energy, and resonance is a powerful remedy. The biggest challenge to homeopathy is scientific verification of the residual resonance of pattern (Bellavite & Signorini, 1995; Pavek & Trachtenberg, 1995; Ullman, 1991, 1995).

A classic biomedical criticism of homeopathy has been that its remedies have not been substantiated by clinical trials. Clinical trials provide standard epidemiological tests of treatment efficacy and effectiveness.[2] Clinical and laboratory research have produced results that support homeopathy; these are reviewed in Ullman (1995) and Bellavite and Signorini (1995). The purpose of clinical trials is to demonstrate meaningful or statistically significant differences between groups of individuals: a control group (or those receiving a placebo) and a treatment group.

Current clinical trial methodology is a recent development, with roots reaching back to the 17th century (Gail, 1996). The ability to demonstrate significant differences did not arise until the development of coherent statistical methodology in the late 19th and early 20th centuries. Clinical trials

---

[2] A treatment may be effective in that it produces a benefit to the patient. A treatment may be efficacious in that it works in killing (for example) cancer cells but it may not be an effective treatment in terms of the patient (e.g., patient has a good chance of dying).

have become the benchmark for efficacy and measurement of the effects of drugs produced by the pharmaceutical industry and are also required by the Food and Drug Administration (FDA) before approval of a new drug for distribution. The validity of clinical trials for testing the efficacy of homeopathic remedies has been questioned because the methodology depends on measuring overall differences of effectiveness and safety in sample populations, whereas homeopathic remedies are prescribed on an individual basis according to a patient's constitution and symptoms.

One important aspect of clinical trials is that outcomes are measured at systematic predetermined intervals. Diseases, symptoms, and the course and timing of recovery are idiosyncratic, and if measured in a group of individuals, a large amount of variation can be introduced. To accommodate this problem statistically, large samples or large differences in measurement between placebo and treatment groups are required. Because of the high costs involved in conducting clinical trials, group sizes are frequently small, requiring large differences to be demonstrated. Nevertheless, there have been clinical trials that have shown the effectiveness of individualized care with respect to symptoms if not to the efficacy of a particular remedy.

A review of clinical trial studies on homeopathic treatments showed positive results for the majority of the studies, about the same proportion found in a similar analysis of biomedical studies (Ullman, 1995). Evaluating the claims of one care model with the analytical arsenal of another may at first appear inappropriate, but rapprochement is possible. Homeopathic care claims can be evaluated scientifically by tailoring biomedical clinical trial methods. Examples of homeopathic clinical trials and laboratory animal studies can be found in journals such as the *British Homeopathic Journal* and The *European Journal of Clinical Pharmacology* and in the leading textbook on homeopathic research (Bellavite & Signorini, 1995).

Educational System: For Licensed Health Care Providers

Since the turn of the 19th century homeopathic study groups and self-taught healers have provided lay treatment for personal use; however, homeopathic practice is legally defined as a practice of medicine and may be practiced professionally only by licensed health care providers, including mid-level practitioners, medical doctors, osteopathic doctors, naturopathic doctors, and chiropractors (see also chapter 4). Six state or national organizations currently offer certification in homeopathic education, but certification in itself is not sufficient to allow one to practice homeopathic medicine legally. Certification cannot serve as licensure; only a degree from a professional medical, nurse practitioner, physician assistant, naturopathic, or chiropractic school can provide the legal means to practice any form of medicine and then only under the authority of a state licensure (National Center for Homeopathy, 1996).

In the United States homeopathic medicine requires 4 years of premedical training followed by postgraduate training in a chosen medical field before one is eligible for licensure as a practitioner. Residency programs in homeopathy are board-certified in three states, and three others are laying the groundwork for their own residency programs. To be board-certified a homeopathic physician must complete 1 year of a residency and at least 6 months of homeopathic training and must pass an exam with a minimal score of 75%. For licensed health professionals, formal training in homeopathy is available in two ways. Professional homeopathic courses on history and philosophy, scientific principles, clinical assessment, the materia medica, diagnosis, and treatment are offered by the National Center for Homeopathy. Alternatively, the medical practitioner wishing to learn homeopathic skills can apprentice himself or herself to a knowledgeable, experienced homeopathic physician for 6 months to 1 year.

DELIVERY SYSTEM: CONTRASTING EXAMPLES FROM PENNSYLVANIA AND NORTH CAROLINA

Generally, homeopathic treatment is provided from a physician's outpatient clinic or office. Private physicians, either medical doctors or doctors of osteopathy, often are board-certified in internal medicine, family medicine, or pediatrics and provide allopathic, osteopathic, and/or homeopathic treatment, depending on what the individual's diagnosis and prognosis require. Preventive care is routinely delivered, and health screening for chronic disease is practiced. Some homeopathic practitioners emphasize family care; others focus on adult health. Few homeopathic pediatricians are in practice (National Center for Homeopathy, 1996); however, guides for homeopathic self-care of children are available (Schmidt, 1996; Ullman, 1992).

The degree of acceptance and delivery of homeopathic care varies considerably across all spatial scales. To elucidate this variation, homeopathic care delivery is compared and contrasted in Pennsylvania and North Carolina. Both states possess major international pharmaceutical and medical industries. However, considerable differences exist in availability and acceptance of homeopathic remedies and treatments.

In Pennsylvania, with a 1995 population of over 12 million (United States Bureau of the Census, 1996b), 13 licensed physicians, 3 veterinarians, 1 nurse practitioner, 2 physician assistants, 2 naturopaths, and 1 chiropractor are listed as practicing homeopaths. Fourteen study groups are spread across the state. In North Carolina, with a 1995 population of over 7 million

(United States Bureau of the Census, 1996b), 2 physicians, 1 naturopathic physician/registered nurse, 2 veterinarians, and 1 chiropractor are listed as practicing homeopaths. Six North Carolina study groups, located in urban centers and the mountains, provide few opportunities for lay people to learn about homeopathy. No study groups or practitioners are located east of Raleigh–Durham, where the largest population of medically under-served live (National Center for Homeopathy, 1996).

Pennsylvania has a history of tolerance of diverse beliefs and practices. Near Harrisburg a large population of German Anabaptist descendants (Amish and Mennonites) reside along with other ethnic and philosophi-cal minorities, such as Hispanic, Asian, and New Age communities. The tradition of tolerance provides a social context in which complementary medicine can be successfully integrated into community life. Amish and Mennonites and other German settlers familiar with homeopathic medi-cine from their homeland form a large proportion of the patient popula-tion of homeopathic physicians. Social and historical structures that allow the development of successful complementary medical practices have not been adequately studied.

In a small community near Harrisburg a family health center was oper-ated by a board-certified internist who was also a board-certified home-opath. He created an interdisciplinary team including a bachelor of science registered nurse (BSRN), a massage therapist, an acupuncturist, a family nurse practitioner certified in homeopathy with a fellowship in women's health, a registered dietitian (RD), a family practice physician, and a phys-ical therapist. Services included well-health care, acute illness care, chronic illness management, mental health counseling, hospital care, health and nutrition education, physical fitness classes, and a nonprofit, organically grown food service. Providers practiced holistically, defined as working with the patient and other providers to find the best methods and treatments to restore wellness. Most health insurance plans covered homeopathic care by a licensed physician or chiropractor. If homeopathic treatment was not indicated, allopathic approaches were practiced, and occasionally, both systems were practiced simultaneously. The regional medical communi-ty's attitude was accepting of homeopathy practice by licensed providers.

A few hospitals across the country provide homeopathic treatment, but not all states have hospital support of homeopathic care. If a homeopathic physician has privileges at a particular hospital, which in most states requires board certification, he or she can have backup depending on hospital policy and the affiliation of other homeopaths. At Holy Name Hospital near Harrisburg, Pennsylvania, board-certified physicians who practiced homeopathy admitted and treated their patients. These home-opaths collaborated with allopathic colleagues to obtain the best individualized care for their patients. This was true for a neighboring osteopathic hospital; however, at a university teaching hospital located within the city, homeopathic treatments were not sanctioned by the hospital board (Borré, 1990–93).

Tolerance of homeopathy in Pennsylvania contrasts with the apathy and rejection homeopathic physicians experience in North Carolina. North Carolina has a large, powerful state medical association that, with the N.C. Board of Medical Examiners, has until recently impeded the legitimate professional practice of most forms of complementary medicine, including homeopathy. The formidable political power these agencies wield led to the case of Dr. George Guess, a family practice physician specializing in homeopathy (*In re Guess*, 1990). The state medical board revoked Dr. Guess's medical license for practicing homeopathy even though he had done no harm to any patient. Two appellate courts overturned the decision, but the state Supreme Court upheld the original decision. Dr. Guess left the state to practice in Virginia successfully, but an outraged public, including several licensed physicians, lobbied the legislature to pass and Governor Hunt to sign a law protecting the right of physicians to practice any form of medicine they consider effective, as long as no harm is done to the patient (Ullman, 1995, pp. 70–72).

If legal means cannot prevent the practice of homeopathy, ostracism and discrimination can be effective in discouraging its practice by instilling fear in physicians. An extreme example of these informal means is reported in Borré's (1990–93) field notes from a 1983 interview with a board-certified, North Carolina–licensed family physician who practiced homeopathy. This physician was incarcerated for practicing homeopathy even without a patient complaint. Consequently, she was admitted to a psychiatric ward and given electroshock therapy with her family's approval. When released, she refused to stop homeopathic practice and subsequently lost her license to practice medicine in North Carolina because of colleagues' complaints.

North Carolina biomedical physicians know little about homeopathy and do not teach alternative therapies in medical schools. A second-year medical student challenged Borré during a lecture on culture and medicine as to whether or not a physician did not have a "moral charge" to educate patients against "wasting their money on quacks" like homeopaths. Ullman (1995, p. 71) noted that "quackery" is best prevented by education of the public, but emphasized that the purpose of education is to allow the public the right to make informed decisions. The appropriate answer for the medical student was to become educated about homeopathy as well as about the patient's illness and then plan with the patient the best treatment, allopathic or homeopathic or complementary. Unless a paradigm shift can occur in medical education, making it truly interdisciplinary, scientific, and collaborative with patients and complementary medicine, these attitudes will be difficult to change.

In contrast to the medical community's response to homeopathy, one North Carolina medical school has acknowledged patients' beliefs in certain forms of alternative health care. One internist brought a local root doctor into the hospital to treat a man who believed he was cursed with a spell. Root doctors, who practice a mixture of syncretic Christian healing, voodoo, and herbalism, are still common in rural North Carolina. One department has instituted the policy of including the chaplain as a member of hospital rounds. The chaplain conducts a religious evaluation of the patient and works with Christian physicians to pray with their patients or address other intrinsic faith and healing issues. Research is being conducted to validate the effect of prayer and religious belief on medical outcome measures (King & Bushwick, 1994). Pentecostalism and beliefs in Christian healing are traditionally strong in North Carolina.

The acceptance of homeopathic medicine in North Carolina is exacerbated by public ignorance, narrow training of physicians, and a politically conservative medical community closely linked to large pharmaceutical companies. These structural characteristics may be true for many communities. A major interesting difference between Pennsylvania and North Carolina lies in the cultural origins and geographic locations of certain populations as well as in the historical and political differences in the establishment of the states. Political and religious tolerance was more narrowly defined in colonial North Carolina than in colonial Pennsylvania. Early settlers who remained in eastern North Carolina were largely Scottish, Irish, and the descendants of slaves. Early Scottish and Irish settlers in south central Pennsylvania were supplanted by the German immigrants and their cultural traditions. When an arthritic nursing home patient in North Carolina requested referral to a homeopathic physician for treatment, no help could be found. Had he requested a Christian, faith-healing physician or a root doctor, many would have been available. Geographic distribution of cultural traditions are part of the social structure supporting the kind of alternative health care that can prosper in a region.

PHARMACEUTICAL AND TREATMENT MATERIALS SUPPORT SYSTEM

Homeopathic remedies are manufactured according to Hahnemann's Materia Medica and more recent formulations by seven major pharmaceutical corporations located in four states. Two West Coast and two East Coast firms distribute wholesale to homeopathic and biomedical pharmacies, health food stores, and physicians. Remedies are available to the public through direct retail sales. These firms also provide educational, research, and technical support to providers, retailers, and the public. Homeopathic Educational Services in Berkeley, California, the largest supplier of educational information, supports research in medical education and clinical trials of homeopathic remedies. Six nationally located homeopathic foundations and organizations provide financial and technical support for research and professional and public education. Directories of homeopathic physicians, study groups, and services are distributed publicly. Two British associations also offer homeopathic support services in the United States.

Boiron Research Institute, located in both California and Pennsylvania, funds qualified scientists to conduct homeopathic clinical trials and other studies to test the efficacy of remedies. The National Institutes of Health (NIH) funds homeopathic research through the Office of Alternative Medicine (see chapter 14). Eleven programs in seven different states and Canada offer homeopathic training to licensed health care providers. Homeopathic dental training and veterinary courses teach diagnosis and treatment of dental problems and animal illnesses. Since 1986 the National Center for Homeopathy has organized formal study groups throughout the country to support self-study by the public and licensed medical providers. The center also offers an annual summer institute to meet the continuing educational needs of licensed providers and others.

LEGAL AND ECONOMIC REGULATION

Only certified and licensed health care providers may practice homeopathy legally within each of the 50 states (see chapter 4). Prescription doses of remedies are dispensed only by registered pharmacists at retail stores. Over-the-counter remedies can be sold anywhere, but pharmacists and vendors cannot prescribe. Individuals with knowledge of homeopathy can prescribe remedies only for themselves and family members. Veterinarians and dentists are allowed to practice homeopathy with certificates from training programs.

One means of economic regulation is accomplished through insurance reimbursement. Many major insurance companies reimburse for homeopathic care provided by licensed providers according to state regulations, state policies, and individual contracts. Medicaid and Medicare reimbursement rules are the same as for biomedical care.

Professional fees, comparable to those of other specialty certification fee structures, are charged for training and certification. Homeopathic board certification entails similar costs to physicians, as do other regulated boards. Certification fees are structured to help regulate health care providers but do not discriminate across general medicine specialties, such as internal medicine, pediatrics, and family medicine.

PUBLIC EXPECTATION: A RENAISSANCE OF HOMEOPATHY

The billion-dollar alternative health industry is the strongest indicator of American interest in seeking care from sources other than biomedicine. Homeopathy is a part of this renaissance of consumers taking control of their health care. Vials of homeopathic remedies are showing up in retail drug and food stores next to the aspirin. Combination homeopathic remedies are marketed to make it easier for the public to choose a remedy on the basis of an illness, not just symptoms. Homeopathic advertising appears on national television and in popular literature. The demand for and enrollment of physicians, other health practitioners, and the public in homeopathic courses and study groups increases annually (National Center for Homeopathy, 1996).

Information about homeopathic training, research, and care is rapidly increasing, as indicated by journals that have debuted in the past few years. *Alternative Complementary Therapies* (1995), *Alternative Health Practitioner: The Journal of Complementary and Natural Care* (1995), and *Alternative Therapies in Health and Medicine* (1994) all include information on homeopathy. Homeopathic Internet websites and listservers are growing in size and number. The largest website of homeopathic information, http://www.homeopathic.com, is that of Homeopathic Educational Services. It offers articles on homeopathy and a catalog of books, tapes, medicines, software, and correspondence courses. Major book chains stock the latest homeopathic self-care books.

CONCLUSION: WHERE WILL HOMEOPATHY RESIDE IN THE 21ST CENTURY?

Clearly, the politics of American biomedicine and that of the complementary medicine movement are unfolding rapidly. Homeopathic medicine appeals to those who reject technocratic approaches to their lives (Davis-Floyd, 1992; Gillett, 1994). In the era of escalating health care costs, most of which is spent on the dying days of our older citizens, homeopathic care is relatively inexpensive and has fewer side effects than conventional treatments. Homeopathic self-care is a popular concept, not only because it can save money but because its philosophy and assumptions parallel recent public awareness of the importance of wellness and preventive health maintenance. Multiculturalism and transglobal communication lead humans to an awareness of other multiple health care systems, which may have some solutions to the problems biomedicine has not solved. The American public will explore these multiple paths until they find their limits.

Undoubtedly, new methodologies of testing homeopathic remedies need development, and funds must be secured to do the clinical research necessary to test both the effectiveness and the efficacy of known remedies in large populations. Research into new remedies will be indicated as better understanding of biophysics develops. Beyond this technical/scientific picture, political structures must be built to support a complementary system of health care. Such a system ideally would be interdisciplinary, patient-oriented, and cost-effective, emphasizing wellness and respect for the individual's body, mind, and soul. Whether or not alternative health care and biomedicine can form one ball of string to focus on the quality of life and the health of the American population will in part be determined in the board rooms of the dominant health care industry. The decision is not wholly theirs, however, because market forces reflecting health awareness and demand for a more effective and human health care system are apparent in the renaissance of homeopathy today.

Narrow paradigmatic medical practice is a disservice to the public and can lead to institutionalization of ignorance. The largest threat to expanding paradigms is the fear of losing control over decreasing economic resources for health care. This is the threat physicians feel from managed care. Fear of losing influence over patients and perceived threats to physician autonomy can lead intelligent and reasonable physicians to become entrenched in biomedical myths. These myths can fuel a dangerous movement within medicine to prevent the whole-ball-of-string paradigm from developing. Current interest in alternative health care systems gives providers an opportunity to establish a new medicine for the 21st century.

PART III

The Changing Medical Marketplace

Healing is a matter of time, but it is sometimes also a matter of opportunity.
—Hippocrates, Precepts I

Part Three examines economic aspects of alternative therapies. In chapter 6, Rena Gordon and Gail Silverstein note that attempts to lower the costs of health care through managed care plans are influencing the way health care is being marketed. Patients, once the target of marketing strategies for biomedical practitioners, have been superseded by managed care plans. Patient-consumers remain the primary market for alternative providers, although insurers increasingly are a factor. Marketing strategies of alternative providers and how they are used to attract patients are discussed. Strategies include advertising, building referral networks, using central referral sources, participating in health and natural products expositions and conventions, and linking with natural and health food stores. The authors address constraints on marketing strategies of alternative practitioners, such as insurance, liability, licensure, and accreditation issues.

In chapter 7, Alan Osborn addresses questions of where alternative providers tend to locate their practice. He presents a case study of the geographic distribution of alternative healers in California, Oregon, and Washington and maps almost 9,000 practitioners by county clusters, or "healthsheds." The greatest absolute numbers of alternative practitioners are found in the largest metropolitan areas, but the practitioner-to-population ratios are highest in less metropolitan or secondary urban areas. Reasons for the latter finding can be related to the types of generalist services alternative practitioners provide, the relatively high incomes of populations in these areas, and/or the amenities provided in these areas.

Childbirth in the United States is an excellent example of how alternative and biomedical practitioners compete in the health care marketplace. In chapter 8, Dona Schneider shows how midwifery has been co-opted and controlled by biomedicine. She traces the history of childbirth from the decline of midwifery and the increasing medicalization in hospital settings to demands from women for alternative practices such as home births and to attempts by the biomedical profession to incorporate such alternatives as nurse-midwives into their practices. Although only a relatively small percentage of babies are delivered by midwives, the percentages vary considerably by geographic area. Interviews with personnel involved in childbirth revealed a consensus that physicians, not midwives, control birth, mainly because of their control of the "money trail." Meanwhile, midwives have become mainstream.

6

Marketing Channels for Alternative Health Care

Rena J. Gordon and Gail Silverstein

One change makes way for the next, giving us the opportunity to grow.
—Vivian Buchen, Welcome Change

Traditionally, medicine has been viewed as a public trust rather than a commodity. Across the nation, medicine increasingly is being reshaped to focus on saving money. Savings have been achieved by employers who were paying double-digit increases in premiums for employee health care and who now provide managed care programs. By 1994 medicine through managed care was a reality for 20% of the nation's population (American Association of Health Plans [AAHP], 1996). Experts estimate that, by the turn of the century, national enrollment in managed care will be over 30%, exceeding 112 million (*Managed Care Digest,* 1995).

The 20% enrollment figure for 1994 is rather conservative because it is based solely on health maintenance organization (HMO) penetration rates. Enrollments in preferred provider organizations (PPOs) and in other types of managed care programs are difficult to track. Therefore, HMO data, although not inclusive of all types of managed care, provide the only available solid representation of enrollment (AAHP, 1996).

There is variation across the country in participation rates in managed care. As shown in Table 6.1, 10 states plus the District of Columbia have 25% or more of residents enrolled in HMOs, 14 states have from 15% to 24.9%, 15 states have from 5% to 14.9%, and 11 states have less than 5%. Highest HMO enrollments are found in Arizona, California, Colorado, Connecticut, District of Columbia, Maryland, Massachusetts, New York,

TABLE 6.1   Managed Care Market Penetration Rates by State, 1994

State	HMO % of Total Population	State	HMO % of Total Population
Alabama	07.2	Montana	02.1
Alaska	00.0	Nebraska	11.2
Arizona	34.6	Nevada	06.1
Arkansas	03.6	New Hampshire	16.3
California	36.9	New Jersey	16.2
Colorado	25.6	New Mexico	17.5
Connecticut	28.3	New York	25.5
Delaware	16.8	North Carolina	08.7
D.C.	01.6	North Dakota	01.5
Florida	00.5	Ohio	19.2
Georgia	08.9	Oklahoma	07.6
Hawaii	23.5	Oregon	35.4
Idaho	01.3	Pennsylvania	23.2
Illinois	18.4	Rhode Island	20.6
Indiana	08.3	South Carolina	04.9
Iowa	04.3	South Dakota	02.9
Kansas	07.1	Tennessee	14.9
Kentucky	11.0	Texas	11.4
Louisiana	08.2	Utah	25.6
Maine	07.2	Vermont	08.1
Maryland	37.5	Virginia	08.7
Massachusetts	40.6	Washington	18.2
Michigan	19.6	West Virginia	00.0
Minnesota	17.3	Wisconsin	26.3
Mississippi	00.3	Wyoming	00.0
Missouri	19.4		
Total	19.7%		

Source: American Association of Health Plans, 1996

Oregon, Utah, and Wisconsin, suggesting a regional pattern with the highest enrollment on the Pacific coast, the Southwest, and the North and mid-Atlantic coast.

This chapter is divided into three sections. The first discusses changes in the ways that biomedical physicians market their practices to patients. The second examines marketing strategies of alternative providers and how they are expanding those strategies to reach an ever-increasing cross-section of the population. The third covers marketing constraints or challenges of alternative providers that are not faced by their biomedical counterparts.

MARKETING STRATEGIES OF
BIOMEDICAL PRACTITIONERS

Physicians and other biomedical health care providers have not typically been in the position of needing to advertise their services or "market" their practices to attract new patients. In fact, historically, there has been widespread criticism of professionals such as physicians who advertise their services through paid media (e.g., billboards and/or newspaper and radio advertisements). Patients, or clients, were attracted through an informal professional referral network among peers. Health care providers would build a practice through social and professional contacts. Until recently, professionals who advertised their services were viewed as suspect by their colleagues and as somehow "faulty" by prospective patients. The mind-set was that "if they were really good, they wouldn't need to advertise for patients."

PATIENT-CONSUMERS

In the past, fee-for-service medicine and indemnity insurance were the predominant approaches to paying for health care. In this approach patient-consumers had the ultimate choice of providers, as long as the health care provider of their choice accepted their type of insurance. It was a rare physician who did not accept most traditional fee-for-service or indemnity insurance plans. Fee-for-service medicine refers to the payment mechanism whereby the provider charges the payer, whether an insurer or the patient directly, for each service provided. The majority of indemnity insurance programs require cost-sharing with the patient, usually requiring that the patient pay 20% of the bill and the insurer pay the balance.

The revolution in health care that has occurred and continues to occur has changed the view of marketing by health care providers. The growing popularity of managed care has probably had the most significant impact on physicians' need to market their practices.

MANAGED CARE PLANS

Managed care plans, including HMOs, PPOs, and other arrangements, have in common the establishment of a contracted or preferred provider network. Managed care abbreviations are defined in Table 6.2. From the standpoint of practice expansion, these managed care plans can have both advantages and disadvantages for the health care provider.

If a provider is in demand by these health plans, his or her mere presence on multiple plans could be enough to provide all the patients that a

TABLE 6.2   Managed Care Abbreviations

FFS (fee-for-service, or indemnity) means payment for each service provided. Indemnity, or traditional insurance, uses the FFS approach; covered persons can use any provider or hospital. They pay a deductible and co-payment, with the insurer absorbing the rest of the fee.

HMO (health maintenance organization) is a health plan that provides coverage of designated health services for a fixed, prepaid premium. The four basic models are (1) group, (2) independent practice association, (3) network, and (4) staff. Some models have physicians on salary who serve only plan members, and members are covered only when they use the HMO's doctors and hospitals. Under the federal HMO Act, an HMO must have an organized system for providing health care or otherwise assuring health care delivery in a geographic area, an agreed-upon set of basic and supplemental health maintenance and treatment services, and an enrolled group.

IPA (independent practice association) is an HMO-type model that contracts with a network of physicians to provide health care services in return for a negotiated fee. Physicians continue in their existing individual or group practices and are compensated on a per capita, fee schedule, or fee-for-service basis. Plan members are covered only when they use designated physicians and hospitals.

MSO (mangement services organization) includes physicians, usually independent practitioners in their own offices, and one or more hospitals. The MSO not only negotiates contracts with third-party payers but also provides management services for the physician offices, including billing and collections, administrative support (which can include hiring and supervision of personnel), and other services.

PHO (physician hospital organization) is an organization composed of physicians and a hospital, which allows them to negotiate with third-party payers as one entity. PHOs are often started and funded by hospitals and seen as transitional organizations in markets that are just entering into managed care arrangements.

POS (point of service) health plan allows the covered person to choose to receive service from either a participating or a nonparticipating provider, with different benefit levels. Plan members usually pay a higher premium and higher co-payments for using nonparticipating providers. The service can be provided in several ways: An HMO may allow members to obtain limited services from nonparticipating providers, provide nonparticipating benefits through a supplemental major medical policy, or use a PPO to provide both participating and nonparticipating levels of coverage and access.

PPO (preferred provider organization) is a program in which contracts are established with preferred providers of medical care. Usually, the contract provides more liberal benefits (fewer co-payments) for services received from preferred providers, encouraging their use. Persons covered are generally allowed benefits for nonparticipating providers' services, usually on an indemnity (fee-for-service) basis with significant co-payments.

provider needs to meet the financial goals of that practice. Provider desirability in managed care plans could be related to geographic location, specialty, quality and reputation, or to the provider's reputation among managed care plans related to appropriate utilization of services (degree of managed care "savvy"). Conversely, if a health care provider is excluded from these preferred provider networks, the population of possible patients available to that provider becomes greatly limited. A patient enrolled in an HMO generally cannot visit a provider who is not on the health plan unless the patient wants to pay for the services out-of-pocket. Some managed care arrangements allow for the patient to see noncontracted providers but at a significantly higher cost to the patient. Frequently excluded from preferred provider panels are physicians who do not meet the previously described criteria indicating a physician's desirability. Osteopaths also are often excluded, as are chiropractors and other alternative health care providers.

To gain advantage in attracting insurance payers, many physicians are aligning with other physician groups and management companies. Contracting with management service organizations (MSOs), independent practice associations (IPAs), and physician hospital organizations (PHOs) creates larger physician groups, which can negotiate higher fees from HMOs as well as relieve physicians of scheduling, payroll, and billing and supply them with medical technologies to improve and track patient health. In some group situations, physicians receive a salary and/or an ownership stake in the group as an incentive to be efficient and generate higher profits.

MARKETING STRATEGIES OF
ALTERNATIVE PRACTITIONERS

The transition from fee-for-service medicine to managed care affects alternative providers somewhat less than allopathic and osteopathic providers because insurance plans do not traditionally cover alternative health care services. Approximately 75% of all services rendered by alternative providers is paid directly by the patient. That cost was more than $10 billion in one year (Eisenberg et al., 1993), almost as much as out-of-pocket hospital costs. These national data also reflect patient payment patterns at a local level. For example, 80% of all services rendered at the clinic of the Southwest College of Naturopathic Medicine and Health Sciences, located in metropolitan Phoenix, Arizona, are paid for directly by the patients (M. Cronin, ND, college president, personal communication [Gordon], February 19, 1996). The relationship between insurance coverage and the availability of a ready panel of patients cannot be overestimated.

PATIENT-CONSUMERS

Typically, alternative health care providers use five types of marketing strategies to attract new patients to their practices. They include (1) advertising, educating-informing through print media, television, radio, and the Internet; (2) building referral relationships with other providers; (3) using central referral sources, such as professional associations, directories of alternative providers, and information hotlines; (4) participating in health and natural products expositions or conventions; and (5) contacting and connecting with natural and health food stores. These five types of commonly used approaches to build a practice are supplemented by an informal word-of-mouth network of referrals from satisfied patients. Amplification of these approaches follows.

Advertising

Alternative providers tend to advertise in publications that are likely to be read by those interested in alternative health care. They target their advertising to this growing audience in such publications as *Natural Health, New Age, Delicious: Your Magazine of Natural Living, Health Store News,* and *Natural Health Shopper,* just a few from a myriad of subscription and free publications published both nationally and regionally. Widespread mass marketing (e.g., billboards and major daily newspapers) are inappropriate media for use by alternative providers because the providers' target population is a fairly specific segment of the general population. Mass media is extremely expensive because of the large number of individuals exposed to it, and the value is wasted if the majority of viewers are not interested in the service. In addition, as with biomedical physicians, mass media advertising does not generally lend itself to public perceptions of professionalism. As the bias against physician advertising decreases and the general acceptance of alternative health care continues to expand, the mass media will become a more important source of advertising to alternative health care providers.

Information and education about natural medicine, an indirect means of advertising or expanding the target population, have made inroads in the national media. On television, for example, Bill Moyers's highly acclaimed Public Broadcasting Service series, *Healing and the Mind,* and the accompanying book (1995), which soared to the top of best-seller lists, as well as Dan Rather's special weekly reports on alternative health practices, captured record audiences. There is much information over the airwaves too: Public Radio International (PRI) presented *The Medicine Garden,* a 1-hour health special series on herbal remedies. The show explores the resurgence of herbal health care through interviews with leading authorities on herbal medicine, including physicians, pharmacologists, botanists, and other scientists. Another radio program, *Natural Alternatives Health Radio Network*, is a weekly, hour-long, ongoing series of short pieces on the folklore, history, and scientific research on specific natural medicines ("Media," 1996). Local programs also are popular and usually feature noted local and national alternative practitioners as guests of the week who make themselves available to answer listener call-in questions.

A relatively new and underutilized source of information on alternative medicine is the worldwide interconnected computer networks on the Internet. There are resources for professionals and others who seek to communicate as well as to gather information about alternative medicine (e.g., see Hancock, 1994; Makulowich, 1994; resource list in chapter 14, this volume). The Internet is emerging as a new medium for advertising and for developing referral networks, the next type of strategy discussed.

Building Referral Networks

The second marketing approach is building referral relationships with other providers, which has been and continues to be an important source of patients for both biomedical and alternative providers. These networks can include referral relationships with other alternative providers as well as with biomedical providers. For example, an acupuncturist can have patients referred through an established relationship with a licensed naturopathic physician or, less often, through a referral relationship with an allopathic or osteopathic physician. Generally, referral patterns among mainstream allopathic and osteopathic providers are developed through interaction with peers in the hospital setting, through relationships developed in professional associations and organizations, and through participation in managed care networks. Because the managed care plan determines who may be used for referrals, the list of contracted providers can substitute for an established referral relationship between two health care providers. Because the majority of alternative health care providers are not on preferred provider panels with managed care plans, they are denied access to possible referral relationships.

The development of referral relationships between biomedical providers and alternative health care providers in the United States is more difficult than among either group of peers, as there is far less interaction professionally. In Britain, where alternative treatments are increasingly supported by the National Health Service, more than 40% of family doctors refer patients for some form of alternative therapy (Jones, 1995). Borkan and his associates (Borkan, Neher, Anson, & Smoker, 1994) conducted a study of mainstream primary care providers in three locations, Washington State, rural New Mexico, and southern Israel, to determine referral patterns of biomedical physicians to alternative health care providers. Their findings indicated no significant differences in referral rates among these varied geographic settings. Fifty-five percent to 77% of the respondents had referred patients to alternative providers at least once during the previous year. These findings could be higher than expected because they include chiropractic referrals for spinal manipulation. The biomedical physicians' decisions to refer patients to an alternative provider were based, in order of frequency, on patients' requests, the synergy between the alternative therapy and the patients' cultural beliefs, patients' lack of response to conventional treatment, and the belief that patients have "nonorganic" or "psychological" problems.

There is a crossover group of physicians composed of allopathic and osteopathic doctors trained in biomedicine who practice holistic medicine (see chapter 13). These physicians are more likely to have referral relationships with alternative providers, as their belief structure tends to go beyond the Western biomedical model.

Certain managed care plans and insurers have developed relationships with alternative providers, either contracting with them directly or allowing biomedical network providers to refer to alternative providers outside the network in appropriate circumstances. As a result of Washington State's new law requiring insurers to cover any licensed provider, Group Health Cooperative in Seattle (a large managed care plan composed of allopathic physicians) has established formalized referral relationships with alternative providers, including acupuncturists and massage therapists. These are new and in some cases tenuous relationships for physicians who are not familiar with the therapies or the providers of those therapies (B. Wolters-Johnson, Alternative Care Coordinator, Group Health Cooperative, personal communication [Silverstein], July 2, 1996). Relationships are starting to become formalized. At Kent Community Health Center Natural Medicine Clinic in suburban Seattle (the first publicly funded alternative clinic in the nation), a naturopath and a biomedical physician work as a team to provide care to county patients at a lower cost (reported on ABC television, January 31, 1997).

In Phoenix, Arizona, the Arizona Center for Health and Medicine is a primary care center staffed by biomedical physicians who practice holistic medicine. The center also offers services such as Chinese medicine, acupuncture, homeopathy, nutritional therapy, and other alternative therapies. Several managed care plans in the Phoenix area, as well as indemnity insurers, cover selected services at the center. One of the unique aspects of the center is its parent organization. It is part of the large Mercy Healthcare Arizona/Catholic Healthcare West system and also receives support from the University of Arizona College of Medicine (Moore, 1995).

Using Central Referral Sources

The third approach commonly used by alternative health care providers to market their practices is participation in national and state associations and organizations, which provide not only referral sources among peers but also publish directories or maintain central referral telephone lines. For example, the American Holistic Medical Association is the professional association for MDs and DOs who practice holistic medicine (see also chapter 13). The organization provides continuing education programs for its members, as well as publishing a national directory of its members (who choose to be listed) by geographic area. The association states that a high volume of calls is taken daily from individuals requesting copies of the directory for a $5 charge.

One may inquire about alternative specialties at state offices, associations or certifying boards for information on individual practitioners or to obtain other referrals. Examples of resources for referrals include the Academy for Guided Imagery, which provides a free catalog and directory of practitioners; the National Center for Homeopathy, which provides an information packet and directory; and the American Association of Acupuncture and Oriental Medicine, which provides information and a referral list of accredited members. Schools that train alternative practitioners and holistic health-related organizations and centers also have directories and can act as referral sources.

Participating in Health and Natural Products Expositions and Conventions

The fourth marketing approach used by alternative providers is participation in segments of the natural products industry that hold major conventions every year in different locations. It is useful to look at this large, diverse industry, first, to examine its size and recent growth; next, to define its components; and finally, to determine how it is employed as a marketing channel for alternative providers. This industry serves the growing number of people who already use or are likely to use alternative practitioners. The customer base has widened to include more than the baby boom generation, appealing also to older people who are looking at alternative health measures and to young mothers in their 20s who want better food for their children (Emerich, 1996). Reasons for the rapid expansion of the customer base, according to industry experts, is that Americans are searching for natural, effective, and safe health care solutions, for more personal control over health care, and for ways to prevent illness.

The natural product industry is big business. According to the 15th Annual Market Overview conducted by New Hope Communications Research of Boulder, Colorado, sales reached $9.17 billion in 1995, an impressive increase of 22.6% over $7.55 billion sales in 1994 (Emerich, 1996), and nearly doubled in just 4 years the 1991 sales of $4.64 billion (Arnold, 1992). Sales growth in dietary supplements, which include vitamins, homeopathy, and herbs, was so strong in 1995 that the stock of publicly traded dietary-supplement companies increased in value by 80%, far exceeding the 1995 increase for the Dow Jones industrial average of 33.5% (Kolata, 1996a).

The natural products industry has three major channels of retail sales: (1) natural food and health food stores, (2) health food chains, and (3) the mass market. In the first channel are 6,600 stores that devote almost all shelf space to natural products, including perishables, dry groceries, prepared foods, bulk food, personal care items, frozen foods, dietary supplements, organic products, books, and housewares. The general distinction between health food stores and natural food stores is that the former receive at least 40% of sales from vitamins, supplements, herbs, and/or personal care items, whereas the latter receive at least 40% of sales from food products. The stores range in size from small and medium health food stores to large natural foods supermarkets. Stores in this channel contribute more than two thirds of total industry sales.

In the second channel are the large health food chains, which focus on vitamins, supplements, herbs, and personal care items, with very little food product. With 2,643 stores in this category, the largest of the three chains is General Nutrition Centers, followed by Great Earth and Fred Meyer.

In the third channel is the mass market, which includes approximately 136,000 mainstream grocery and supermarket stores across the nation. It is estimated that from 60% to 80% of mainstream stores carry some natural products. Also included are drugstore chains and mass merchandisers such as Kmart and Wal-Mart. Not included in any of these channels or their sales figures are multilevel marketing and mail-order sales of natural products, which gain much of their sales in rural areas and through the World Wide Web.

Retailers in the natural products industry come to expositions and conventions to be educated about new products and about healing. The number of products introduced at these shows has doubled in the first half of the 1990s (Emerich, 1996). In 1996 an estimated 4,000 to 5,000 new natural products, not including supplements, were introduced at expos. The number of supplements also is growing daily. It is estimated that 80% of the products available now were not even in existence 4 years ago (Picozzi, 1996). This proliferation of products presents a challenge for the industry and for the consumer. Expos are held to help educate the industry on these products.

Three organizations—Natural Products, National Nutritional Foods Association (NNFA), and Whole Foods—each sponsor two annual conventions. In 1996, for example, the Natural Products Expo West in Anaheim, California, drew 20,000 convention attendees in the spring, and the Expo East show in Baltimore, Maryland, also attracted thousands. The NNFA-SW Trade Show in Austin, Texas, and the NNFA-NW Trade Show in Seattle, Washington, also drew large numbers of participants.

Samples, demonstrations, and product literature help vitamin and other buyers keep up with the explosion of information. Leading practitioners, research scientists, and writers in alternative health care, including respected physicians Andrew Weil, Larry Dossey, and Deepak Chopra, give keynote addresses and participate in forums and seminars. Alternative practitioners attend and/or leave cards and materials at show booths and interact with peers and attendees, all of which help develop referral networks. Although the natural foods and health industry is big business, those in the industry are reminded of the fact that they are involved in healing. People go to health food stores to buy products, but they also go to become well (Anderson, 1996). Over 90% of customers make their first visit to a natural products store because they are experiencing a health crisis (Emerich, 1996, p. 22).

Connecting with Natural and Health Food Stores

The fifth approach of marketing is through natural and health food stores, which contribute more than two thirds of total industry sales and traditionally have been and continue to be an important avenue for marketing alternative therapies and for building referral relationships. Common to these stores are written materials on holistic health, herbs, vitamins, supplements, and alternative therapies. There are racks, bulletin boards, file cabinets, and even libraries containing a wide variety of information and educational materials available to interested consumers.

Although natural and health food stores are sources of referrals to alternative providers, they are careful regarding specific referrals, making no recommendations, representations, or endorsements of any individual or entity for a customer who inquires about an alternative health care provider. These stores are more consumer-oriented than are the big chain stores (the second channel), which would direct a customer who asks for a referral to listings in the telephone book. The natural and health food stores make available a range of opportunities for referrals, from a bulletin board for posting business cards or a file box with names of alternative practitioners to a printed list with a table of contents identifying the types of health care professionals listed. A southern California landmark is Mrs. Gooch's Whole Foods Market, founded in 1977 on a "commitment to offer the highest quality natural foods, related products, services and information which optimize and enrich the health and well-being of the individual as well as the planet" (from a 1996 brochure). At an upscale Mrs. Gooch's market in Beverly Hills, customers requesting names of practitioners are given a copy of a 24-page list of alternative health care providers by specialty, prefaced by the following statement:

> We at Mrs. Gooch's know that it is sometimes difficult to find alternative health care practitioners. With that in mind, we have compiled this list of health care professionals who specialize in various areas of holistic health care. This information is provided only as a convenience to you, our patrons.
>
> Whether you choose a practitioner from this list or not, you should do a thorough investigation of anyone you might select to use and satisfy yourself of the person's ability to perform the services you desire to have performed. We cannot take responsibility for the quality of services rendered by any of the facilities or practitioners contained within.
>
> Additionally, we strongly urge you to interview any practitioner with whom you are considering treatment. . . . To assist you in your investigation, you may call various associations and/or Boards listed herein and inquire about the individual's professional standing within the association and/or Board. They may be able to refer you to other sources of information to assist you in your investigation.
>
> Your health is your responsibility, and through education and research you can join forces with various health professionals and fulfill your health care requirements in ways that suit you as an individual.

INSURERS

Alternative health care means good business for insurance companies. Growing consumer demand, as well as less costly therapies, are appealing to the insurance industry. Several insurers have taken pioneering steps in covering selective therapies.

There are currently 15 insurance companies, including the giant Mutual of Omaha, that cover physician Dean Ornish's diet and wellness plan for preventing and reversing heart disease. The cost of Dr. Ornish's program (approximately $5,500) may be seen as a sound investment if it enables patients to avoid $15,000 angioplasties and $40,000 bypass operations. Estimated savings from Dr. Ornish's low-tech program is $6.50 for every dollar Mutual of Omaha has spent. Eventually, they could save up to $20 for each dollar spent (Cowley, King, Hager, & Rosenberg, 1995). American Western, based in California and available in several western states, covers numerous alternative therapies, including acupuncture, massage, hypnotherapy, and others.

As of January 1, 1996, insurers in Washington State are mandated to cover any licensed provider. This includes alternative therapies that are licensed in the state (acupuncture, chiropractic, naturopathy, and massage; see chapter 4 on state licensure). This law is likely to result in a significant increase in consumers' access to alternative therapies, because the services will now be covered by indemnity insurance and managed care plans. Many states will be watching and evaluating Washington's experience as they draft their own legislation related to insurance coverage of alternative therapies. Despite major progress in insurance coverage of alternative therapies, most alternative health care is still paid for by the patient directly. This in itself limits the possible number of patients. Also, providers are not supplied with a "captive" panel of patients, such as those enrolled in a managed care plan.

MARKETING CHALLENGES FOR ALTERNATIVE PROVIDERS

Alternative health care providers face numerous marketing barriers not experienced by their biomedical colleagues. One major disadvantage is the still common lack of insurance coverage for alternative therapies. Physicians and insurance companies have legal and economic incentives to consider the viability of alternative health care. They include cost savings and threat of suit for negligence. In respect to cost savings, Mutual of Omaha reports it saves about $6.50 for every dollar it spends covering nonstandard treatment, such as a diet-based alternative to surgery for heart disease. In respect to threat of suit for negligence, an executive of a leading private health insurance company said that the reason for the lack of insurance coverage was the fear of malpractice suits (D. J. McIntyre, vice president, Blue Cross and Blue Shield of Arizona, personal communication [Gordon], September 9, 1994). In an ironic twist, patients who have not been given the option of receiving alternative treatments in their health plan are beginning to sue insurance companies.

INSURANCE AND LIABILITY ISSUES

A recent move in New York State could set a national precedent. A national coalition of physicians and patients is building a case in New York against insurance companies that do not reimburse policyholders for alternative health care. The 1994 New York State Alternative Medical Practice Act gives broad powers to physicians by allowing them to prescribe any care that "effectively treats human disease" (as determined by the physician). However, physicians are finding that they may prescribe a treatment, but their patients are not getting reimbursed for it. The Foundation for the Advancement of Innovative Medicine (FAIM) calls for insurance carriers to cover policyholders for alternative medical treatments such as acupuncture or nutritional counseling. They also want coverage for experimental treatments awaiting government approval and off-label use of prescription drugs. They have taken their case to the New York State Department of Insurance, the official body that arbitrates insurance regulation.

An expert on preventing malpractice litigation notes that those who do not offer viable alternatives to potentially toxic prescription drugs can open themselves up to lawsuits. By not meeting the legal definition of informed consent, patients who have not been offered alternatives have begun to sue for negligence ("Unconventional Claims," 1995, p. 27).

Procedures considered experimental are usually not included in insurance coverage. The March 1996 ruling of the FDA has stamped acupuncture needles as legitimate medical tools, like syringes and scalpels. This decision has taken acupuncture needles out of the experimental category. Practitioners of the technique and makers of the needles have met with major health insurers on reimbursement issues ("Acupuncture insurance?" 1996).

In an article on gaining insurance coverage for alternative therapies, Colgate (1995) studied the strategic processes by which three alternative therapies—chiropractic, acupuncture, and biofeedback—gained acceptance. Because third-party reimbursement is viewed as a significant indicator of acceptance by both the biomedical community and the public, she examined the insurance coverage given each therapy and summarized the data into a concise set of acceptance criteria by both the biomedical community and the insurance industry. Of the 18 insurers included in the study, 9 covered chiropractic; 8, acupuncture; and 11, biofeedback.

The acceptance or reimbursement criteria for alternative therapies are

- ability to fit into the existing diagnosis-based system;
- willingness to be viewed as a complementary, not competing, therapy;
- willingness to follow the generally accepted biomedical model of professionalism by providing education standards and accreditation, professional licensure, and documented clinical practice guidelines; and
- availability of adequate and appropriate research.

The results of her study indicate that chiropractic, acupuncture, and biofeedback each have achieved at least moderate success in obtaining third-party reimbursement. Each therapy targeted a market niche: lower back pain by chiropractic, acute pain and detoxification by acupuncture, and acute pain management by biofeedback. Also, each therapy met criteria expected by the biomedical health care and insurance systems of this country. These moderate successes can be useful as a guide for other new treatment or therapy attempts to gain third-party reimbursement.

Licensure and Accreditation Issues

In addition to providing services still largely not covered by insurance, licensure and accreditation are additional hurdles faced by alternative health care providers when determining how best to market their services. Although biomedical physicians can market themselves as "board certified" or as graduates of well-respected medical schools, many alternative health care providers do not have these credentials. Currently, 11 states license naturopathic physicians (for specific states see chapter 4) and acupuncturists are licensed in far more states. This may in part be a result of the interest and training of some biomedical physicians in acupuncture.

The licensure of alternative health care providers is something of a two-edged sword. Naturopathic doctors (NDs) in Washington State, for example, can be licensed and can advertise themselves as graduates of Bastyr University in Seattle (one of three recognized naturopathic training programs in the United States), but they also are more likely to practice in Washington State. According to an official at Bastyr, it is difficult for a new graduate of their program to establish a solo practice in Seattle, where there are already a large number of practicing naturopaths. A graduating ND may be more successful practicing in a state that does not license these providers because of less competition and therefore a more easily established niche in the market. If a state does not license a particular type of health care provider, it affects the scope of practice of that provider, who can, however, still practice to a limited degree.

Many alternative therapies do not have accrediting bodies such as those that exist for biomedical practitioners. Patients seeking such providers must be especially cautious and take a "buyer beware" approach. Unless the recommendation for a provider is by word of mouth from a trusted friend or relative, the consumer has fewer commonly recognized methods of assessing an alternative provider's credentials than would be available for a more mainstream provider.

CONCLUSION

The revolution in health care is just beginning. Increasing consumer demand as well as economic pressures on the health care system are likely to move alternative health care continually closer to the mainstream. The Washington State experiment has much to teach other states in terms of merging the biomedical and alternative models into one system, at least from a reimbursement perspective. Many alternative providers in Washington view the new law as a two-edged sword: respectability brings complications.

The availability of insurance coverage for their services promises to increase their patient volume, lend an increased air of mainstream respectability to alternative health care, and increase the reimbursement of providers (potentially making a career in these specialties more appealing to many). On the down side, incorporation of insurance payments into a medical practice brings with it a whole array of additional complications, such as use of specific billing forms, coding, and possibly prior authorization of services. Billing clerks have to be hired, and the practice no longer operates on a simple cash basis. Life suddenly becomes more complicated for alternative health care providers as they join the economic mainstream of American health care.

Movement toward this mainstream is likely to expand referral sources for alternative health care providers. As discussed in this chapter, public awareness of alternative health care is growing as patients obtaining services from these providers are seeing the results they are looking for. Insurance company decisions are driven by economics and consumer demand. More and more, consumers are requesting company benefits administrators to include alternative medicine in their coverage, and they are having some success. A case in point is Blue Cross of Washington and Alaska, which decided to offer coverage of alternatives after customers bombarded the company with that request (Griffin, 1995). As insurers expand their coverage of alternative health care services, biomedical physicians and alternative health care providers will develop referral relationships that previously did not exist—if not by choice, then by virtue of appearing on the same "contracted provider" list.

Although there are certainly biomedical physicians who see the value of alternative therapies for certain patients and in certain circumstances, such therapies also can be seen as a threat to biomedical providers. Says Joseph Pizzorno of Bastyr University in Seattle, "Fundamentally, if you can teach people how to take care of themselves, they don't need doctors, and that's seen as a threat by many people" (Egan, 1996).

Alternative health care providers will continue to face marketing challenges that biomedical physicians do not face. In many parts of the United States, alternative health care providers are not readily available. Because states vary greatly in the types of providers that are licensed and schools that train alternative providers are not well known, credential and licensure issues will continue to present difficulties for alternative providers in marketing to mainstream consumers. In light of the lack of commonly accepted standards of care in alternative medicine, consumers should be well informed about their options in both alternative medicine and biomedicine. The appeal of alternative therapies has grown far beyond the original small niche of young, educated consumers and will continue to grow as the baby boom cohort ages. It has still to achieve its full economic potential. Over the course of the next several years, advertising in natural and health food stores could be supplemented or replaced by participation of alternative providers on "preferred provider" lists, particularly if cost savings as a result of using alternative therapies continues to be documented.

7

The Regional Distribution of Alternative Health Care

Alan Rice Osborn

What region of the earth is not full of our calamities?
—Virgil

This chapter discusses how alternative medical services are distributed across space and why it is important to understand this distribution. The chapter begins with a brief discussion of the processes of diffusion and distribution, then specifically looks at how practitioners of alternative medicine in the western United States are distributed. Using a case study, the relationship between population and the number of alternative practitioners in an area is examined, a relationship that is not as simple as it first appears. Although the greatest number of practitioners is found in the largest urban areas, the highest ratio of practitioners to population is found in less metropolitan or secondary urban areas. Reasons for this pattern are discussed, and recommendations for future research are made.

Very little is known about why alternative practitioners choose to locate in a particular place. Why are some kinds of alternative services available in one place and not in another? What factors affect the distribution of alternative medicine? Is it possible to predict where alternative practitioners will locate?

The way diseases spread and evolve are studied so that changes in health care needs can be understood and planned for. It also is important to study how different types of health care are distributed, as well as how their distributions change; which areas are medically underserved; and what changes are seen for the future. During the past 30 years geographers have examined the distributions of many different aspects of the United

States health care system—clinics, hospitals, physicians, and patients (Gesler, 1991). But the role of alternative health care in the United States (and in other developed countries) has been largely ignored (Fulder, 1986; Gesler, 1988).

Alternative practitioners and their patients have been almost invisible, at least in terms of officially compiled health and health care statistics (Fairfoot, 1987; Satin, 1988). Although there has been considerable research to the contrary (McGuire, 1988; O'Connor, 1993), all too often both patients and practitioners have been regarded as naive, eccentric, and willful: "The conventional view of nonorthodox health belief and practice is that at best it is marginal, used only by folks who are poor, uneducated, or socially isolated, and perpetrated by practitioners who are either fraudulent or simply ignorant" (Clouser & Hufford, 1993, p. 101).

Rather than studying alternative medicine, authors "have taken either the perspective of medical orthodoxy, producing tirades against the [alternative] movements, or have upheld alternative therapies, penning polemics accusing detractors of shortsightedness and self-interest" (Moore, 1990, p. 265).

In the United States, "about a third of all American adults use unconventional medical treatments" (Campion, 1993, p. 282), and well over $10 billion per year is spent on alternative health care (Campion, 1993; Eisenberg et al., 1993). Alternative systems of healing "hold a strong collective appeal for individuals who mistrust or are somehow disenchanted with mainline medicine" (Cassedy, 1991, pp. 147–148) and are an important part of the health care "lifeworld" (Gesler, 1991, p. 164) of a significant proportion of the population.

Alternative health care has become popular, widely available, and an increasing part of American health care. How and why something that is so widespread, that affects so many people, and that has such "an enormous presence in the United States health care system" (Eisenberg et al., 1993, p. 251) operates certainly needs to be explored and examined. By better understanding the distributional characteristics of alternative health care in the United States today, we can gain insight into how it functions within the health care system and how it may function in the future.

DISTRIBUTION AND DIFFUSION

Why are some types of alternative medicine confined to a specific place or culture while others are widespread? Answering this kind of question leads to a deeper understanding of how the elements of the health care system work and interact.

Distribution is largely a matter of diffusion, the way that cultural elements spread from their point of origin. Every system of health care has "important spatial components" (Shannon & Dever, 1974, p. 89), and different types of health care develop different types of distributions.

As an example, consider acupuncture. Acupuncture was introduced to the United States about 1825 (Zwicky, Hafner, Barret, & Jarvis, 1993, p. 39) but was regarded by Western medical practitioners for more than a century as contemptible and "ridiculous" (Inglis & West, 1983, p. 11). Beginning with a warming political climate between the United States and China in the 1970s, attitudes began to change: "eminent American physicians . . . had to admit . . . they had been impressed by what they had seen" (Inglis & West, 1983, p. 11). In the past few years many American physicians have been eager to try acupuncture (Kao & McRae, 1986). Today there are thousands of acupuncturists (and practitioners of related therapies) in the United States (Wardwell, 1994).

The process by which acupuncture became a part of our health care system demonstrates several different types of diffusion. It originally came to the United States with an immigrant group, a process called relocation diffusion (ideas spread when a group of people migrate or relocate), but cultural and legal barriers prevented its wider acceptance. In the 1970s it spread, first from a small number of "eminent physicians" in major medical centers to the broader medical community in a process called hierarchical diffusion (ideas spread from more important persons or larger places to less important people and places). After that it traveled through the general population, largely spread by the media, through contagious diffusion, so called because the process is similar to the way a contagious disease spreads.

In addition to diffusion, one other concept that is helpful in understanding distribution is Central Place Theory. In general, it can be expected that the larger an urban area, the greater the variety of goods and services it will have (King, 1984). This seems intuitively reasonable—it would be very surprising to find large numbers of highly specialized medical services in a small town or to find that a major city did not have a great diversity of services available. However, there are many exceptions to this pattern. Historical background, transportation, economic and governmental factors, cultural and political barriers, and the physical environment can all affect the kind and variety of services available in any given place.

By being aware of the processes by which ideas and innovations spread, of the different ways that ideas can diffuse, and of the ways that goods and services tend to be arranged, we can begin to understand why different types of health care tend to have different distributions.

PROBLEMS OF DEFINITION AND INCLUSION

As discussed in chapter 2, one of the knottier problems encountered in any study of alternative health care is the difficulty of deciding what is "alternative" (see Table 2.1). Another major difficulty is deciding which modes of healing to include (see Table 2.2).

There is also the problem of the health care "underground." Many nonprofessional providers of health care do not advertise their services. Some are culturally based within ethnic or immigrant groups (e.g., Gypsies, Mexican Americans, people from isolated areas in the Appalachian and Ozark Mountains) (McClenon, 1993). Others are found primarily in educated middle-class groups (e.g., religious healing, the home birth movement, hypnosis) (McGuire, 1988; O'Connor, 1993). In either case it is extremely difficult to study these practitioners because they operate outside typical medical and legal channels. Finding them can be "arduous" (Perrone, Stockel, & Krueger, 1989, p. xii).

Alternative health care modalities that have significant numbers of practitioners in the western United States are included in the case study: Chinese medicine and related therapies, including acupuncture, acupressure, shiatsu, and reflexology; chiropractic; holistic medicine; homeopathy; and naturopathy.

CASE STUDY: CALIFORNIA, OREGON,
AND WASHINGTON

Relatively little research has been done on the distribution of alternative practitioners in the United States. All previous studies, with the possible exception of Monmonier (1971), have looked at the distribution of alternative health care services either within a particular state (Gesler, 1988; Marshall, Hassanein, Hassanein, & Marshall, 1971; Thaden, 1951), or within a portion of a state (e.g., a city, county, or group of counties) (Hassinger & Hastings, 1975; Osborn, 1990; Yesalis, Wallace, Fisher, & Tokheim, 1980). This case study was designed to see how alternative health care services are distributed throughout a larger area. By focusing on health care "catchment areas" composed of aggregated county units, patterns can be seen that would be hard to perceive at local, state, or national levels.

Data were collected at the county level in California, Oregon, and Washington. Practitioner locations were compiled by using the most recent available telephone directory for each county. Telephone directories were chosen as the source of location data for four reasons: (1) they are available for all counties in the region; (2) they are a reliable source of data on practitioner locations (Mattingly, 1991); (3) specific state licensing is not required for many alternative health care modalities, and state agencies frequently list home addresses, mailing addresses, and the addresses of people no longer in active practice; and (4) there are no dominant national or regional organizations for most alternative health care practitioners; in some cases, there is more than one national organization. Practitioner listings from such organizations, under the circumstances, are of dubious value. Although it is true that "telephone directories have been shown to be biased against representation of lower socioeconomic status households" (Kviz, 1984, p. 801), this should not be a significant problem in this study in which the focus is on the popular and well-known types of practitioners discussed previously.

Using a total of 82 different telephone directories, 8,928 practitioners were located. Because people cannot be expected to limit their health-seeking behavior on the basis of county boundaries (Monmonier, 1971, p. 123), the county data were aggregated, state by state, into health care "catchment areas," that is, into regions within which most individuals can be expected to seek and receive most of their health care. This process is analogous to drawing watershed boundaries for streams and rivers, and the health care catchment can be thought of as a kind of "healthshed."

However, determining health care usage boundaries is more an art than a science (Harner & Slater, 1980; Morrisey, Sloan, & Valvona, 1988; Rowley & Baldwin, 1984; Stimson, 1981). For this study the catchment area in urban regions is assumed to be equal to the 1990 United States Census Metropolitan Statistical Area (MSA) (Morrisey et al., 1988). For less urbanized and rural areas, directory service (Yellow Pages) coverage areas are used as the catchment area boundaries (Rowley & Baldwin, 1984).

Several points concerning study methodology should be noted. First, licensing procedures vary, and not all of the alternative practitioner categories are found in all three states (see Table 4.1). For example, naturopaths are not licensed and cannot legally practice (at least, not as naturopaths) in California.

Second, there is nothing to prevent a practitioner from advertising in more than one category. As a worst-case example, an individual could conceivably list himself or herself simultaneously in the acupressure, acupuncture, chiropractic, homeopath, holistic practitioner, naturopath, reflexologist, and shiatsu practitioner categories. Further, a single practitioner can also list himself or herself more than once within a single category—for example, a chiropractor could advertise herself as "Smith, Jane, Chiropractor," "Jane Smith Chiropractic" and "JSC Chiropractic Corporation." Of course, multiple listings cost more, so there is a financial disincentive against this practice; however, a great many health care professionals apparently find the investment worthwhile. Efforts were made to prevent duplicate listing, but it is quite likely that some errors were made, so the total number of practitioners included in this study may be slightly inflated. On the other hand, nonprofessional alternative health care practitioners (e.g., Mexican *curanderas*, faith healers, herbalists) are not included, so the total number of these alternative practitioners in California, Oregon, and Washington is probably much larger.

Finally, although the aggregation process for catchment areas was generally as described above, certain exceptions were made, based on propinquity, observation, and previous experience with the region. For example, Riverside and San Bernardino Counties (the California Desert Counties catchment (see Figure 7.1)) are within the Los Angeles–Anaheim–Riverside Consolidated Metropolitan Statistical Area (CMSA) but outside the Los Angeles MSA; despite large communities along the Los Angeles and Orange County boundaries, these counties are for the most part rural and sparsely populated and so are separate from the Los Angeles area catchment.

RESULTS

California was divided into 11 catchment regions using the aggregation procedure described above (Figure 7.1). California's population is concentrated in four areas: San Diego and Los Angeles in southern California and the San Francisco Bay area and Sacramento in northern California. A basic understanding of Central Place Theory indicates that the greatest number of practitioners should be located in the largest urban areas, and in fact this is the case. However, the ratio of practitioners to population within the catchment areas shows a different pattern. The highest ratio of alternative practitioners to population is found in the Central Coast catchment: Monterey, San Benito, San Luis Obispo, Santa Barbara, and Santa Cruz counties.

Oregon was divided into 10 catchments (Figure 7.2). Oregon's population is concentrated in the Willamette Valley and in the Portland MSA. Again, based on our understanding of how goods and services tend to be arranged, the greatest number of alternative practitioners should be in the largest urban area. This is the case; the overwhelming majority of alternative practitioners (55%) are concentrated in the Portland area. However, once again, the ratio of practitioners to population within catchment areas shows a different pattern. The highest ratio is found in the Central Oregon catchment: Crook, Deschutes, Jefferson, and Wheeler counties.

Washington was divided into 12 catchments (Figure 7.3). Washington's population is concentrated in the Seattle MSA and south of Puget Sound. As before, the greatest numbers of alternative practitioners are in the

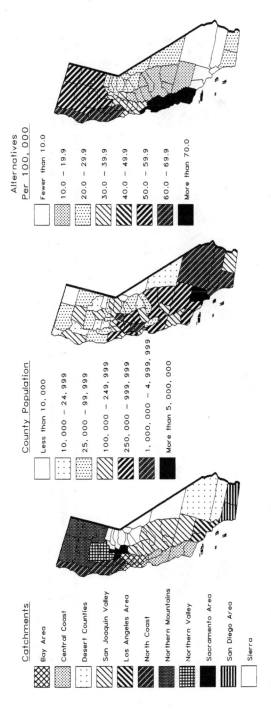

Catchments

Bay Area

Central Coast

Desert Counties

San Joaquin Valley

Los Angeles Area

North Coast

Northern Mountains

Northern Valley

Sacramento Area

San Diego Area

Sierra

County Population

Less than 10,000

10,000 – 24,999

25,000 – 99,999

100,000 – 249,999

250,000 – 999,999

1,000,000 – 4,999,999

More than 5,000,000

Alternatives Per 100,000

Fewer than 10.0

10.0 – 19.9

20.0 – 29.9

30.0 – 39.9

40.0 – 49.9

50.0 – 59.9

60.0 – 69.9

More than 70.0

FIGURE 7.1   Regional distribution of alternative practitioners in California. California was divided into 11 health care catchments. The map of population by county shows that the highest population concentrations are in Los Angeles, in southern California, and in the San Francisco Bay area. The map of alternative practitioners per 100,000 shows that the highest ratio of alternative practitioners is in the Central Coast catchment.

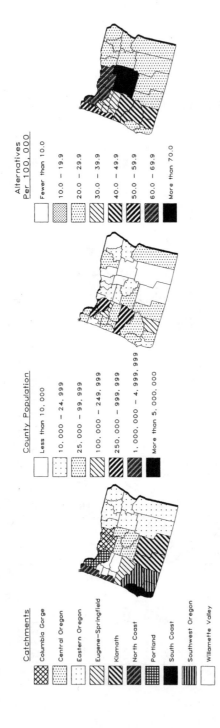

FIGURE 7.2 Regional distribution of alternative practitioners in Oregon. Oregon was divided into 10 health care catchments. The map of population by county shows that the highest population concentrations are in Portland, Eugene–Springfield, and the Willamette Valley. The map of alternative practitioners per 100,000 shows that the highest ratio of alternative practitioners is in the Central Oregon catchment.

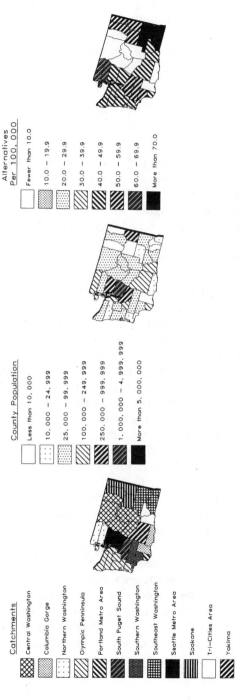

Catchments

Central Washington
Columbia Gorge
Northern Washington
Olympic Penninsula
Portland Metro Area
South Puget Sound
Southern Washington
Southeast Washington
Seattle Metro Area
Spokane
Tri-Cities Area
Yakima

County Population

Less than 10,000
10,000 – 24,999
25,000 – 99,999
100,000 – 249,999
250,000 – 999,999
1,000,000 – 4,999,999
More than 5,000,000

Alternatives
Per 100,000

Fewer than 10.0
10.0 – 19.9
20.0 – 29.9
30.0 – 39.9
40.0 – 49.9
50.0 – 59.9
60.0 – 69.9
More than 70.0

FIGURE 7.3   Regional distribution of alternative practitioners in Washington. Washington was divided into 12 health care catchments. The map of population by county shows that the highest population concentrations are in Seattle and in the Spokane area. The map of alternative practitioners per 100,000 shows that the highest ratio of alternative practitioners is in the Southeast Washington catchment.

113

largest urban areas, but again, the map of the ratio of practitioners to population per catchment region shows that the highest ratio is not. The highest ratio of alternative practitioners to population is in the southeastern Washington catchment: Adams, Asotin, Benton, Garfield, Walla Walla, and Whitman counties.

DISCUSSION

If only numbers of alternative health care practitioners are looked at, the regional distribution appears to be very easy to explain: the greater the population, the greater the number of practitioners. Only when the ratios of practitioners to population are mapped do we see that the relationship is more complex. In each state the highest ratios are found not in the largest urban areas but in what might be called secondary urban centers. What does this distributional pattern mean?

Research has shown that the more "metropolitan" an urban area, the greater the specialist-to-population ratio; that is, the greater the urban population, the greater the number of specialist health care practitioners. On the other hand, the less metropolitan an urban area, the greater the general-practitioner-to population ratio; that is, the smaller the urban population, the greater the number of general practitioners and primary care physicians. This is the pattern seen in the maps of alternative-practitioner-to-population ratios. In terms of their distribution, alternative practitioners seem to be much more like general practitioners than they are like specialists. From this it can be inferred that alternative practitioners function more like general practitioners than specialists within the health care system.

Place—the social, economic and demographic characteristics of a particular location—also must be considered when analyzing the distribution of health care delivery (Gesler, 1991, p. 167). There are two such characteristics that the central coast of California, central Oregon, and southeastern Washington have in common that suggest why these areas have such high practitioner-to-population ratios. First, all three have large enough populations to support some metropolitan amenities but are small enough to avoid the disadvantages of major cities. Second, all three are resort and vacation areas. Such places have their problems, of course (e.g., absentee land ownership, high seasonal transiency, high burglary rates), but they have extremely high visual, recreational, and environmental amenities.

For both alternative practitioners and their patients, this pattern of distribution may be evidence of the "equity refugee" phenomenon—people leaving large cities for smaller, less costly metropolitan areas (Hamel & Schreiner, 1990). This also can be a case of "lifestyle refugees": people who are "fed up with crowds, pollution . . . and expensive houses" and have decided, for economic or personal reasons, "to get away from cities" (Fost, 1990, p. 47) to places they believe are more congenial.

Whether the pattern reflects the equity or lifestyle refugee phenomenon, there appear to be two plausible interpretations of these results. Alternative practitioners may be more likely than the general population to locate in high-amenity secondary urban areas, or it is conceivable that the residents of these places demand more alternative health care than does the general population. At this point it is not possible to say which of these is true, but it can be said that alternative health care practitioners are present in significant numbers in these secondary metropolitan areas in the western United States, and that they are providing a service that people in these areas want and are willing to support.

CONCLUSION

Alternative medicine today is not "marginal, used only by folks who are poor, uneducated, or socially isolated" (Clouser & Hufford, 1993, p. 101). Many of the consumers of alternative health care are educated, middle-class individuals who can afford to pay for whatever kind of health care they choose (McGuire, 1988; O'Connor, 1993). Studying how alternative health care practitioners are distributed can bring some understanding to the social and economic context in which this phenomenon is taking place.

This study has shown that, in California, Oregon, and Washington, the highest alternative practitioner-to-population ratios are found not in major cities or in rural areas but in high-amenity, relatively nonmetropolitan urbanized regions. This finding has at least two important implications.

First, the fact that the distribution of alternative practitioners is similar to that of general practitioners implies that alternative practitioners are functioning within the health care system as generalists—that is, in a manner similar to that of primary care physicians and general practitioners. Second, because relatively large numbers of alternative practitioners are choosing to locate in certain areas of California, Oregon, and Washington, there must be a market there that can support them. Further research will be necessary before the social and demographic nature of this market can be understood and before such questions as who are the consumers and why do they choose alternative medicine can be answered.

Future research can be directed at answering these and many other important questions. For example, can the results of this study be generalized, or is this region atypical? Are alternative medical services spreading into new places, and if they are, by what kinds of diffusion processes (e.g., contagious, hierarchical, etc.)? If alternative practitioners are functioning as primary health care providers, is it because there is a shortage of Western biomedical practitioners in the area, or do patients use them in addition to standard medical care? Does increased cooperation between alternative medicine and biomedicine affect the distribution of alternative practitioners? Is alternative medicine becoming elitist—have alternative practitioners abandoned both the rural and the urban poor to work with the wealthy?

This is a time of transition, moving from a period in which there was a single, nearly universally accepted health care paradigm to a period of pluralism and diversity. The study of the distribution of alternative medicine is a rich and productive area for research. A greater understanding of how our health care system is evolving will be gained by seeking answers to these questions.

8

Demand for Alternative Therapies: The Case of Childbirth

Dona Schneider

Innovation is resisted by individuals who are unwilling to risk the status they have achieved and jealously guard their own job against any change.
—William T. Brady

Although efforts by physicians to control the medical marketplace were quite successful for more than half a century, some alternative therapies simply could not be snuffed out. The social and economic ramifications of denying patients access to alternative therapies crystallized over the past few decades as physicians who denigrated a patient's wishes to seek the help of an alternative care provider often lost that patient as a client. More recently, third-party payers began to recognize that many patients could be satisfied with the less expensive treatments provided by alternative care providers. Given that some alternative therapies were not going to fade away, physicians responded by (1) co-opting these therapies into the mainstream and (2) controlling patient access to them by dominating third-party payer panels.

Today it is no longer uncommon for a mainstream practitioner to refer patients to an acupuncturist for pain control, to a chiropractor for common neck and back problems, or to a midwife to act as the birth attendant for a normal vaginal delivery. Indeed, a few physicians have trained as acupuncturists themselves. Others have found that sharing office space with a chiropractor can be lucrative because patient referrals can go both ways. And across the United States, many obstetricians and prepaid health care systems have found that hiring a midwife to help with heavy patient loads and to reduce the stress of night calls is a far less expensive solution to their problems than taking on a new physician. Not only do providers save money in salary and the costs of malpractice insurance, they have the added benefit of being perceived as progressive, as responsive to women's demands. In other words, hiring a midwife for an obstetrical practice provides a good marketing advantage. Indeed, midwifery is a perfect example of how alternative therapies become co-opted and controlled by mainstream health care practitioners, a need that became more critical for the traditional obstetrical establishment as the baby boomers moved through their childbearing years.[1]

This chapter has two purposes. First, it provides a general overview of the history of childbirth alternatives in the United States. Second, it describes not only the struggle between obstetricians and midwives to control the childbirth marketplace but also that between women and the traditional medical establishment over the right of women to make choices about their own childbirth experiences.

A CENTURY OF CHILDBIRTH ALTERNATIVES

Childbirth is an event that reflects social norms, the socioeconomic status of the mother, and the location at which the birth takes place. At the turn of the century, most births in the United States took place at home. Hospitals of the time were places people went to die, not to give birth. A female relative or friend might have attended the laboring mother unless she had the means to pay a physician to come to the home. The number of midwives was on the decline, and midwifery services were no longer readily available except in rural areas and the ethnic immigrant sections of cities (Litoff, 1978).

The decline of midwifery by the beginning of the 20th century was the result of a highly successful campaign waged by physicians to portray midwives as dirty, backward, and poorly trained. State legislatures responded to these charges by passing laws restricting the practice of midwifery. In fact, many states demanded licensure of midwives even before they required physicians to be licensed (Ehrenreich & English, 1973). As the pool of midwives dried up, physicians filled the void as birth attendants, challenging the socially accepted norm that pregnancy and childbirth were natural processes. Over time, pregnancy and childbirth came to be viewed as conditions requiring expert medical management (Wertz & Wertz, 1977).

---

[1] Much of the information in this chapter was obtained from anonymous interviews with obstetricians, midwives, directors of midwifery training programs, and hospital and birthing center administrators.

By 1920, physicians solidified the perception that they were the keepers of the latest in childbirth technology by offering in-hospital painless childbirth, or "twilight sleep." Women of means could be admitted to maternity wards, minimize the pain of childbirth through the use of anesthesia, and remain in the hospital for lengthy periods to recover from the experience. Poor women and those living far from hospitals that provided maternity services remained dependent on home delivery.

By midcentury, hospital birth became the social norm for all but the poorest of women and those living in remote areas. Antibiotics that could cure specific infections were available. Blood transfusion techniques were developed and blood banks established to lessen the dangers of postpartum hemorrhage. Anesthesia techniques were developed that were safer and that allowed the laboring woman to be conscious during delivery. Oxytocic drugs, agents that promote rapid labor, were developed and counteracted with the slowing effects of anesthetics. As a result of these technologic advances, maternal mortality in the United States dropped from 70 per 10,000 in 1930 to 7 per 10,000 by 1955, and neonatal mortality slipped from 32 per 1,000 in 1930 to 20 per 1,000 by 1955 (Wertz & Wertz, 1977). This dual success of the medical establishment, providing both safety and relief of pain in childbirth, all but made the midwife extinct.

One less successful side effect of the biomedical model for childbirth was that the miraculous event became mechanized and institutionalized. The laboring woman was admitted to the hospital like any other patient, given an enema, and shaved of all pubic hair. The woman was then moved to a labor room, given an analgesic and scopolamine, and when she had sufficiently progressed, moved to a delivery room and placed flat on her back on a table. The woman's legs were strapped into stirrups above her body in the lithotomy position, a position selected by obstetricians for ease of access to and control of the perineal area rather than for ease of delivery by the laboring woman. Often, a fetal monitor was attached, an intravenous line inserted, and anesthesia administered. Episiotomy, a surgical incision of the vulva to prevent tearing during delivery, was routine. If there were complications, the patient would be taken to the operating room for a caesarean section. After the placenta was delivered, the patient was sutured and again transferred, this time to a recovery room. Finally, the childbirth experience was complete when the new mother was transferred to her room on the maternity ward.

During this entire experience, fathers were expected to remain in a hospital waiting room. After the infant was cleaned and placed in a bassinet in the nursery, the father was allowed to view the child through a glass window. It was not uncommon for the father to hold the child for the first time only after he had taken the new family home, which was often 10 days to 2 weeks after the traumatic event (Litoff, 1986).

With the passage of Medicaid in the 1960s, even the poorest American women had access to physician-assisted in-hospital delivery. Mainstream medicine had forged the perception that childbirth was now safer than ever because all women had access to the best technology for both themselves and their new infants. Yet some women and a few physicians began to question the assumption that pregnancy and childbirth required medical management and intervention (Bradley, 1974; Chabon, 1966; Dick-Reed, 1959). The women's movement encouraged them to demand control of their bodies (Frankfort, 1972; Rich, 1977; Rothman, 1982; Ruzek, 1978). Paternalistic mainstream medicine was rejected as the norm for pregnancy and childbirth by sympathetic physicians and parent groups who claimed that home birth and midwives as birth attendants were both safe and preferable (DeVries, 1985; Rooks & Haas, 1986; Stewart & Stewart, 1979).

GRASS-ROOTS DEMANDS FOR CONTROL OVER CHILDBIRTH ALTERNATIVES

The women's movement may have begun the process of empowering women to take control of their bodies, but the number of women demanding childbirth alternatives rose during the 1970s simply because the baby boomers were entering their childbearing years. Traditional in-hospital delivery under the care of a physician was not acceptable to all birthing women. Some chose home birth, others sought a midwife-attended birth, and a select few demanded both. Traditional physicians did not react favorably to either possibility.

The movement to return to home birth in the United States began in California. A male midwife, Norman Casserly, was arrested for practicing medicine without a license in 1971. His arrest, conviction, and appeal brought publicity to home birth and led a growing number of women to rally for birthing alternatives.

Some women, especially obstetrical nurses, knew that women wanted their husbands with them at delivery, that they wanted to bond with their babies before they were whisked off to the nursery, and that they questioned whether episiotomies were really necessary. Some of these women agreed to serve as the birth attendant for friends or relatives who refused to submit to physician in-hospital delivery. Their willingness to serve became established in the home birth movement, and they became known as lay midwives. In many states these women could face criminal prosecution for practicing medicine without a license. In other states "granny" and frontier midwives had long been acknowledged as serving the needs of rural communities and did not face the same sanctions (Schrom Dye, 1983). Contrasts among states were stark, reflecting the lack of basic services in some regions and the availability of high technology in others. If hospital services for childbirth were available, the medical establishment and the legislatures they influenced assumed that they should be used.

The American College of Obstetrics and Gynecology (ACOG) responded to the demands for alternatives in childbirth with a policy statement proclaiming that home birth was a form of child abuse and neglect (ACOG, 1975). Mainstream medicine, specifically obstetrics, had a monopoly on childbirth that it was not going to give up easily. The statistics on the safety of the biomedical model for childbirth were well established, and women who demanded less were viewed as irrational. It was even suggested that women who gave birth at home by choice should be prosecuted.

The 1970s saw a rise in the number of specialty-trained physicians and more hospitals offering maternity services than ever before. At the same time, the baby boom demand for childbirth services began to decline, and by the end of the decade competition for births became serious business. Although advertising for patients was still considered unethical during that era, physicians and hospitals knew that if they offered special services, word would quickly spread and they would have a competitive edge for attracting new patients. Some obstetricians offered their pregnant patients Lamaze classes, the medical establishment equivalent of "natural childbirth" that could be adapted to hospital routine.

In response to the complaint that the childbirth experience in the hospital was cold and unfeeling, hospitals removed restrictions that prevented husbands from being in the delivery room and allowed mothers to bond with their babies before sending them off to the nursery. Some progressive physicians agreed to "try" to deliver the mother of her baby without an episiotomy. Mainstream medicine was firm, however, about keeping childbirth in the hospital. Physicians, who were still primarily male and trained in the technological imperative, saw no reason to respond to women's demands they believed would compromise safety—births without fetal monitoring and with a midwife rather than a physician in attendance at normal vaginal deliveries (ACOG, 1979). The fact that lay midwives were becoming licensed in some states and the fact that epidemiologic studies showed that midwives had excellent outcomes for home births did not influence their beliefs (Mehl, 1977; Weitz & Sullivan, 1985).

Most, but not all, women were satisfied with the new in-hospital options available for the birthing experience. The home birth movement would not die; and a new entity, the free-standing birthing center with certified nurse-midwives (CNMs, nurses endorsed as appropriately trained by the new American College of Nurse-Midwives) as attendants began to spring up in the late 1970s (Committee on Assessing Alternative Birth Settings, 1983). Rather than lose business to birthing centers and other hospitals that might be viewed as more progressive, some hospitals hired CNMs for their own staffs (Declercq, 1992; Kohler, Bellenger, & Whyte, 1990). In some cases, hospitals attempted to buy out free-standing facilities. In others, they tried to put the competition out of business with in-hospital birthing centers. This competition for births was demonstrated by the increase of in-hospital, midwife-attended births from 0.6% in 1975 to 3.4% in 1989. Midwife-attended not-in-hospital (home and birthing center) births remained stable for the same period (USDHHS, 1994).

VITAL STATISTICS

Differences in the use of childbirth alternatives by place of delivery, attendant, and race of the mother also can be shown by the use of vital statistics. On the national scale, 4.4% of Black women and 3.1% of White women had their babies delivered by midwives in the hospital setting (USDHHS, 1994). Reasons that more Black women were delivered by midwives in hospitals might be third-party payment agreements or the lack thereof, or residence patterns where Blacks were more likely to deliver in inner-city environments where CNMs were on the staff of "progressive" or teaching hospitals. On the other hand, only 0.24% of White and 0.03% of Black women were attended by CNMs at birthing centers (USDHHS, 1994). These low numbers also make sense as, in 1990, many birthing centers were located in suburban areas and their services were not covered by insurance. The requirements that clients have personal transportation and could self-pay may have precluded many women, especially Black women, from seeking their services.

Of interest is the fact that a larger percentage of Black than of White women were denoted in United States statistics as attended by a physician at home births in 1990 (USDHHS, 1994). Research has shown that this is a data artifact rather than truth (Schneider, 1986). Often, women who deliver at home prematurely are transported to a hospital, where the birth certificate is then completed by the emergency room physician. Rather than having a physician-attended birth at home, these women were likely to have had unattended births. As Black women are statistically more likely to deliver prematurely, these data artificially reflect increased physician at-home deliveries.

Table 8.1 lists the number of live births and the percentage of those births attended by physicians and midwives by United States census areas. In 1990, 3.9% of all live births in the United States were attended by midwives, up from 2.9% in 1985 and 1.8% in 1980. On the regional level the largest percentage of midwife-attended births occurred in the West; the smallest percentage occurred in the Midwest.

TABLE 8.1   Live Births in United States, 1990, by Census Area

U.S. Census Area	No. of Live Births	% Attended by Physicians[a]	% Attended by Midwives[a]
United States	4,158,212	94.95	3.92
Region			
Northeast	792,999	95.07	4.42
Midwest	945,843	97.59	1.35
South	1,409,380	94.50	4.03
West	1,009,990	93.01	5.78
Division			
New England	201,173	93.46	5.96
Middle Atlantic	591,826	95.62	3.89
South Atlantic	700,285	91.94	5.78
East South Central	236,374	96.65	2.45
West South Central	472,721	97.23	2.23
East North Central	675,512	97.41	1.21
West North Central	270,331	98.02	1.67
Mountain	242,829	93.36	5.87
Pacific	767,161	92.90	5.75

[a] Columns do not total 100% as some births were unattended or attended by persons other than physicians or midwives.
Source: U.S. Department of Health and Human Services, 1994, *Vital Statistics of the United States 1990: Vol. 1. Natality.* Hyattsville, MD: National Center for Health Statistics.

As regional data are highly dependent on the areal units aggregated, it is prudent to examine more than one geographic scale to look for pattern. The lower part of Table 8.1 includes census division data (i.e., smaller aggregates of states). Of interest is the fact that the division data now show a quite different pattern from that revealed by the regional data. Specifically, the largest percentage of births attended by midwives in 1990 occurred in New England; the third largest percentage, in the South Atlantic. Divisions of the West (Mountain and Pacific) show as second and fourth, respectively, in terms of percentage of midwife-attended births. The smallest percentage occurred in the East North Central division, a subcategory of Midwest. Indeed, all four Midwest subdivisions accounted for the bottom ranks.

State level data yield even more information. For example, the percentage of midwife-attended births in 1990 ranged from a low of 0.03% in Nebraska to a high of 12.08% in Alaska. State-level data for percentage of midwife-attended births by quartiles are found in Figure 8.1. The pattern cannot be explained as an urban-rural dichotomy or by minority distributions. It more likely reflects the marketplace, that is, changes in the willingness

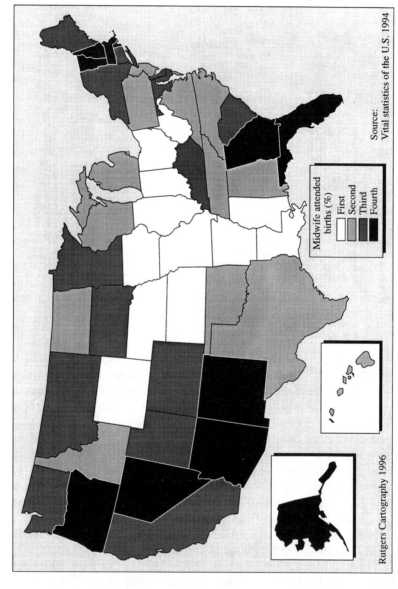

Rutgers Cartography 1996

Source:
Vital statistics of the U.S. 1994

Midwife attended births (%)

First
Second
Third
Fourth

FIGURE 8.1 Percentage of midwife-attended deliveries by state, 1990 (quartiles). From *Vital Statistics of the United States, 1994.*

of third-party payers to cover alternatives in childbirth as these services are less costly than traditional in-hospital obstetric care. Otherwise put, it might be a reflection of a bicoastal pattern of managed care that was far less prevalent in the central portion of the United States during the early part of the 1990s.

THE FUTURE OF MIDWIFERY

The data on childbirth reflect a slow but growing acceptance of midwives as birth attendants over the past two decades, a reversal of the trend seen at the beginning of the century. But has the status of midwifery really changed? Has midwifery truly become mainstream? To answer these questions, the views of 15 practicing obstetricians and midwives, business managers in birthing centers and hospitals, directors of midwifery training programs, and representatives of national organizations, such as the National Association of Childbearing Centers and the American College of Nurse Midwives, were elicited. Their views may not be representative of all midwives, but they do give us clues as to the status of midwifery today and where the profession is headed as we approach the year 2000.

The tone of these interviews might be summed up by the quip of one midwife who noted, "It is lucrative to care for the sick. Just follow the money trail and you will find the power." Indeed, the childbirth business is no exception to this rule. If you follow the money, from payers to service providers, it is clear that physicians hold the power over childbirth, not midwives.

There are several reasons that this is true. One is that the baby boomlet generated by the baby boomers is over, and the competition for births has become cutthroat (De Witt, 1993). Professional societies for physicians, such as the American Medical Association and the American College of Obstetrics and Gynecology, hold large numbers of dollars for lobbying. They have the ability to influence the way payments are distributed for health care and childbirth services covered under programs such as Medicaid. These societies influence state-mandated legislation. In some states, for example, a minimum number of births is needed to maintain the licensure status of facilities that provide birthing services. In others a minimum number of births also is needed for facilities to successfully compete for third-party payment contracts, for licensure to provide high-risk birthing services, and to provide a pool of births for the training of medical students and interns, family practice and obstetric residents, physician's assistants, and future midwives. To guarantee this minimum number of births and also to guarantee their incomes, physicians and hospitals have hired midwives for their own staffs, purchased midwifery contracts from birthing centers and private providers, and actively sought out positions on provider panels to guarantee third-party payment contracts.

In contrast, midwives have had limited success in negotiating directly for third-party payment. One of the roadblocks they have faced is that midwives are low-volume providers. Another is that they are not considered primary care providers by payers, a definition created by the medical establishment and designed to exclude all non-MD providers. In order to practice, then, a midwife usually agrees to employment in a hospital, a birthing center, a health department, or a physician practice. In all these situations the midwife works under the auspices of a physician, and the bill for her services is generated by the employer, the primary care provider, under contract with the third-party payer.

This situation was well characterized by the director of one midwifery program in the Northeast, who said:

> Midwives are naive. We hold a respectable portion of the market share of births, but when you can't bill directly for your services, you are at a distinct disadvantage. Unfortunately, midwives have not yet learned how to negotiate. They need to demand to be made a partner in physician practices and to demand a share in the profits.

Another said,

> The system is corrupt. The hospitals bill Medicaid under a physician's name so they can get maximum payment for the job done by the midwife. HMOs capitate and subcontract their birthing services to OB [obstetric] groups that utilize midwives for these births. There will be no real changes until Medicaid cleans up its act.

If you ask how midwives are faring in this shuffle, the answers you get are mixed. Physicians are still split on whether there should be a role for midwives (Young & Drife, 1992). There are midwives fighting for hospital privileges in many states, for licensure in others. Yet in 1995 the National Association of Childbearing Centers had 135 free-standing childbirth centers staffed by CNMs, as full members of the organization, and an additional 110 centers under development. The membership of the American College of Nurse-Midwives reported an active membership of over 5,000 in 1995, up from almost 3,600 in 1994. Clearly, the roadblocks to practicing midwifery are not deterring persons from entering the profession or from opening birthing centers. They are, however, providing limits on the types of services midwives can offer. For example, a midwife can rarely practice on her own, as the costs of malpractice insurance for a midwife in solo practice are prohibitive (Gordon, 1990; Patch & Holaday, 1989). This limits most midwives to service under the auspices of a physician's practice, a birthing center practice, or a hospital-based or health–department based practice.

Roadblocks within the profession also are falling. In 1994 the American College of Nurse-Midwives asked its members to vote on whether nursing should be a pre- or co-requisite for obtaining certification as a midwife. The membership voted to accept non-nurses with appropriate educational backgrounds in the sciences for midwifery training. The mechanism for training and certifying non-nurse midwives is now in place, and the number of certified midwives is certain to increase.

In the short run, the increase in the number of midwives should pose a major conflict with physicians as the fight over who gets payment for a limited number of births heats up. It may prove a boon to third-party payers, however, as competition should force the cost of childbirth down. In the long run, some providers will fall by the wayside. To survive, providers will have to be creative and flexible, offering more bells and whistles to potential customers and better cost packaging to payers (De Witt, 1993). Whether physicians can retain control in a market glutted with midwives, birthing centers, and third-party payers demanding cuts remains to be seen.

Has the status of midwifery changed? Has midwifery become mainstream? The answer to both questions is emphatically yes. Maligned at the turn of the century, midwives fought back by becoming professionalized, setting standards for their own training and certification (Reid, 1991). Recent epidemiological studies show that their services yield good results (Durand, 1992; Heins, Nance, McCarthy, & Efird, 1990). Today midwives are respected as birth attendants, although they have not been able to get payers to agree that their time is worth as much as that of a physician. Nor have they been able to loosen the control physicians have on midwifery, restricting their hospital privileges and their ability to directly receive third-party payments.

Midwifery also has become mainstream; that is, it has been co-opted by the medical establishment as a marketing strategy and as a means of controlling provider costs. Midwives serve as birth attendants with the sanction of physicians in their private practices, in the hospital setting, and in free-standing birthing centers. They serve as home birth attendants for women who refuse to be hospitalized and may be the only health care professionals serving many rural areas (Bastian, 1993; Lucas, 1993; Taylor & Ricketts, 1993). Today midwives account for a market share of births that can no longer be ascribed to a fringe element demanding alternatives to physician-in-hospital birth.

In 1995 more than 94% of CNMs attended births in hospitals, 12% served in birthing centers, and 7% attended home births (a total of more than 100% reflects the fact that some midwives worked in more than one setting). The fact that midwives serve in these settings, as well as in physician practices (all of which are the domain of biomedicine), shows that the profession has become mainstream.

CONCLUSION

This chapter has presented the argument that there are patterns to the acceptance of alternative therapies as mainstream. Specifically, biomedical physicians hold the power in the health care marketplace and have for more than a century. This mainstream medical movement resists the use of alternative therapies unless it becomes clear that there are marketing advantages to co-opting that therapy into their ranks. By co-opting alternative therapies, biomedicine is able to directly control therapies that threaten to develop on their own, challenging physician control of the medical marketplace. Means of direct control include limiting the practice of an alternative therapy to providers with specific training and/or licensure and to those who work under the auspices of a physician or mainstream medical facility and limiting the ability of alternative care providers to obtain direct payment for their services. Indeed, physicians as gatekeepers for health care services, including access to alternative therapies that might be covered under health insurance contracts, remains the current paradigm. It seems likely that mainstream medicine will continue to co-opt alternative therapies that can provide acceptable services for patients at lower rates unless and until that paradigm is changed.

PART IV

The Culture Complex

*Some people eat with a knife and fork, others with chopsticks, and still others
use their fingers. . . . To each of us, of course, our way of doing things
is the right way. This would not matter so much if it were not for the
complications of the "missionary syndrome," which leads us to try to
persuade other people to abandon their ways and take up ours.*
—*Marston Bates*

Part Four turns our attention to the cultural complex that lies behind
health care–seeking behavior. In chapter 9, Jill Hyatt and Mary Hale
discuss social and cultural aspects of alternative therapies. Their discussion concentrates on shamanistic healing, one of the "alternative: ethnic"
practices listed in the scheme established in chapter 2. For each of four
groups—African Americans, Hispanic Americans, Native Americans, and
Asian Americans—Hyatt and Hale provide a wealth of detail on their beliefs
and belief systems and on who uses such specific ethnic systems or practices as rootwork, *curanderismo*, medicinal plants, or acupuncture. Although
data are often sparse, the authors conclude that these forms of alternative
practice thrive in many communities throughout the country.

In chapter 10, Clarissa Kimber makes a case for focusing on the household medical system when examining people's interactions with both
alternative and biomedical practitioners. A key element is consideration of
the wide variety of dyadic relationships established between clients and
providers. She illustrates the usefulness of the household medical system
concept by showing how households of German extraction in the hill country of Texas use a range of practitioners and practices, including "herb doctors," midwives, bone setters, chiropractors, medicinal plants, faith healers,
and medical doctors, drawing on northern European, Mexican, and Native
American traditions.

In chapter 11, Joan Koss-Chioino reviews therapeutic relationships in
psychology, psychoanalysis, medicine, and allied health disciplines and in
the cross-cultural literature. She introduces a very different model of relating

between healers and clients, one that structures the healing process in alternative practices. She offers as an illustration the healing relationship and healing process in *Espiritismo,* a traditional cult-religion in Puerto Rico and elsewhere in Latin America. This analysis is intended to contribute to a general goal of redefining the healing process to include a spiritual component because these more traditional triadic healing practices are widespread in the United States, especially among ethnic minority and immigrant communities.

9

Social and Cultural Aspects of Alternative Therapies

Jill M. Hyatt and Mary M. Hale

> *To live sacred lives requires that we live*
> *at the edge of what we do not know.*
> *—Anne Hillman*

In the recent national study of alternative medicine use in the United States that has been mentioned earlier in this book, researchers reported that 34% of the 1,539 adults surveyed reported using at least one unconventional therapy in the past year, and a third of those saw providers for unconventional therapy (Eisenberg et al., 1993). Extrapolating from their results to the United States population, the researchers in this study report that an estimated 425 million visits were made to unconventional health care providers by Americans in 1990. This estimate exceeds the approximately 388 million reported visits to all primary care physicians in the United States for the same year.

Researchers in this study also report that, contrary to the beliefs of many alternative health care providers, use of alternative medicine is not limited primarily to narrow or marginal segments in American society. The study reports that rates of use ranged from 23% to 53% in all sociodemographic groups considered. The study, conducted by researchers at the Harvard Medical School and published in the *New England Journal of Medicine*, found that the highest rates of use of alternative medicine were reported by non-Black persons from 25 to 49 years of age who had relatively more education and higher incomes (Eisenberg et al., 1993). Among people age 25 to 49 surveyed by the study, 38% reported use of at least one form of alternative medicine, compared to 33% in younger groups and 27% in older groups. Among African Americans surveyed in the study only 23% reported use of one or more forms of alternative medicine, compared to 35% in other racial groups.

Significant income and education differences were also noted in the study: 44% of those having some college education reported using one or more forms of alternative medicine, compared to only 27% of those with no college education. Of those with incomes above $35,000, 39% reported using one or more forms of alternative medicine, compared to 31% of those with incomes below $35,000. The study also notes that no significant differences in use were found on the basis of sex or insured status.

The results of the study cited above provide a useful overview of alternative medicine use in the United States and, as its authors note, indicate that its use is much higher than previous studies suggest. In addition, the study helps to dispel the notion that use of alternative medicine is limited primarily to poor, uneducated, minority, and marginalized segments of society. At the same time, however, the study has a number of shortcomings (some of which are openly acknowledged by its researchers) that limit the representativeness of its results to the entire population, and to racial and ethnic minority populations in particular.[1] In the sections that follow we address some of these shortcomings through discussion of alternative medicine practices and shamanistic healing systems in general, also focusing on the practice of such systems among several ethnic minority populations in the United States. Specifically, we discuss the alternative medicine beliefs and practices among African Americans, Mexican Americans and other Hispanic Americans, Native Americans, and Asian Americans in some detail. Our focus, then, is on the alternative cross-cultural category set out in chapter 2.

---

[1] There are five major shortcomings to the *New England Journal of Medicine* study that are pertinent here: (1) the definition of "unconventional" medicine and limited numbers of therapies covered in the survey; (2) exclusion of non-English-speaking respondents from the survey—a total of 97 respondents were excluded from participating on this basis; (3) exclusion of households without telephones, shelter populations and other homeless persons, and institutionalized populations; (4) exclusion of 96 respondents from participation in the study because of cognitive or physical incapacity, and underrepresentation of respondents with poor health; only 3% of those surveyed reported that they were in poor health, based on a 5-point scale of perceived health status; among those 3% reporting poor health, 52% reported using unconventional therapy; and (5) the underrepresentation of certain minority groups in the sample (e.g., African Americans comprise over 12% of the U.S. population but only 9% of the respondents surveyed; and Hispanics comprise nearly 9% of the U.S. population but only 6% of respondents surveyed).

ALTERNATIVE MEDICINE PRACTICES
AND SHAMANISM

Although all alternative medicine practices are not part of shamanism, the racial and ethnic groups explored here are regarded by many as shamanistic in their traditional healing practices. Shamanism is an externalizing belief system; that is, problems or illness are thought to originate from spiritual or other outside sources and can be diagnosed from such sources as well (McClenon, 1993). In a recent report to the National Institutes of Health (1994), the following descriptions are offered of shamans and shamanism:

> A *shaman* is a type of spiritual healer distinguished by the practice of journeying to a non-ordinary reality to make contact with the world of spirits, to ask their direction in bringing healing back to the people and the community. . . . The journey is a controlled trance state that practitioners induce by using repetitive sound (drums, rattles), or movement (dancing), and occasionally by ingesting plant substances (e.g., peyote or certain mushrooms). . . . Shamanic practices define healing broadly; not only are people to be healed of their spiritual and psychic wounds, but shamans also attempt to heal communities, modify the weather, and find lost objects. Many traditional shamans are also skilled in . . . herbal practices. (p. 95)

Shamanic healing is practiced worldwide and has roots in much European, African, Asian, and Native American folk practice; currently it is gaining popularity among non-native urban Americans as well. Hispanic American traditional healing systems also contain certain aspects that may be described as shamanistic in nature.

AFRICAN AMERICANS

This section begins with a discussion of the belief system underlying traditional African American medicine and continues with a discussion of the literature on its continued practice.

Beliefs/Belief System

Hoodoo, voodoo, and *rootwork* are all terms used to refer to a wide variety of traditional African American medical, religious and magical beliefs and practices. Kerr (1993) notes that hoodoo can be traced to West African religions and that the word *hoodoo* "is thought to have diverse West African derivations, in particular `juju' (meaning conjure), but may also be an adulteration of voodoo" (p. 609). Kerr identifies both similarities and differences between voodoo and hoodoo, noting that "hoodoo is a more generalized term than is voodoo and may be applied equally to complex magical practices or simple medicinal practices" (p. 609). Fishman, Bobo, Kosub, and

Womeodu (1993) describe voodoo as a religion "characterized by a belief in certain laws, medical practices, taboos and rituals that serve as a powerful force for maintaining cultural identity in some African American sub-groups" (p. 164). Rootwork is the term that "generally described the traditional medical system practiced by African Americans, particularly those living in inner city and southern rural areas" (Fishman et al., 1993, p. 164). The term comes from the idea that plant roots can be used to cast spells. For purposes of simplicity this term is employed here to refer to a variety of hoodoo, voodoo, and rootwork beliefs and practices.

One central feature of the rootwork medical belief system is the division of illnesses into two main categories: natural and unnatural. *Natural* illness is attributed to a lack of harmony in the physical or spiritual world and to an imbalance in the blood. Illness results when blood is "too sweet or bitter, too high or too low, and too thick or thin" and is believed to be caused by dietary and/or lifestyle excesses (Fishman et al., 1993, p. 163). A variety of herbal and dietary remedies are used to treat imbalances in the blood. Yellow root is used to "bitter" blood that is thought to be too sweet; sulfur, molasses, poke greens, sassafras tea, and catnip tea are all used to thin or purify the blood. Beet juice is ingested to treat blood that is low, and drinking garlic water or applying lemon juice or vinegar externally to the face are all treatments for blood that is too high (Snow, 1993). *Unnatural* illness occurs "when one has fallen victim to a hex, curse, or spell (magical causes)," and it is believed to be caused by the consumption of food contaminated (i.e., cursed or hexed) with the eggs of snakes, frogs, or spiders; victims often believe that "the animal is growing under his skin and is causing symptoms of burning skin, rashes, pruritus, nausea, vomiting, and headache" (Fishman et al., 1993, p. 164). In such cases, the family will usually consult a rootwork practitioner. As Fishman and her colleagues note, rootwork practitioners are referred to by a wide variety of terms, including the old lady, spiritualist, conjurer, hoochi coochi man, reverend, bishop, prophet, and voodoo priest.

Who Uses Rootwork and Why

Research data suggest that belief in rootwork is more common among low-income, less educated, working poor African Americans (Snow, 1993) and that its practice is most common among those living in inner cities and southern rural areas (Fishman et al., 1993). There are no normative data and little empirical data in the literature describing the "typical" rootwork user or the extent of its use among African Americans; ethnographic research consists primarily of case studies describing how it works (Kerr, 1993).

The literature on rootwork and African American ethnomedicine in general reveals considerable debate among researchers on the subject as to the reasons for its survival and continued practice. In the epilogue to her book, *Walkin' Over Medicine,* Loudell Snow (1993) tells her readers:

> If the reader comes away with anything from this book, I hope it will be that the traditional ways of healing are still to be found because they serve a purpose. They allay the physical ills of the body, of course, but they heal spirit and mind and heart as well. . . . They offer empowerment to those who, on the surface, have not much power at all. (p. 279)

In a review of her work, Fox (1995) summarizes Snow's view in the following manner: "traditional African American ethnomedicine persists despite access to [biomedical] care because it is a form of community empowerment" (p. 416). Fox takes Snow to task for what he sees as her failure to address such obvious issues as income; insurance status; ability to pay for medical services and prescription drugs; past experiences of pain, humiliation, and discrimination in dealing with conventional (and overwhelmingly Anglo American) medical practitioners and institutions; and the important influence these issues have on African American health care choices. The explanation for the persistence of traditional African American ethnomedicine may be a combination of all of the above. Certainly, religious faith in God as a source of healing power can offer a sense of empowerment to those who believe. In addition, preservation of African American traditions such as rootwork can serve as a source of cultural pride and, in that sense, can be empowering. To argue, however, that traditional African American ethnomedicine persists primarily as a matter of faith, cultural pride, and empowerment is to underestimate greatly the value of those factors that Fox offers as explanations for the persistence of traditional African American healing practices such as rootwork.

HISPANIC AMERICANS

Census data from 1990 indicate that Hispanics are the second largest and fastest-growing minority group in the United States. Mexican Americans are the largest segment of this population group, comprising approximately 63% of all Hispanic Americans (Wright, 1990). The focus of this section, therefore, is on the Mexican American system of folk medicine. This is followed by a brief discussion of the traditional healing methods practiced among the Puerto Rican and Cuban populations.

Beliefs/Belief System

Curanderismo, from the Spanish word *curar* (to heal), is the Mexican American system of folk medicine and healing. Because most *curanderismo* healers are middle-aged and older women, the feminine form, *curandera,* is employed throughout this discussion. *Curanderismo* combines elements of medieval Spanish medicine and Catholicism with elements of Native American medicine and healing (Gomez & Gomez, 1985; Marsh & Hentges, 1988). Maduro (1983) describes *curanderismo* as a "coherent world view of healing." One commonly held belief is that the mind and body are inseparable. This contrasts sharply with what has been referred to by some as the dichotomization of mind and body historically seen in conventional Western medical practice. This belief in the inseparability of the mind and body informs the understanding of illness and its causes in the system of *curanderismo*. For example, it is believed that illness may result from having experienced strong emotional states. Such illnesses include *bilis*, which is caused by *rabia* (rage); *susto* (soul loss), caused by extreme fear or sudden fright; *envidida*, resulting from extreme jealousy or envy; and *tristeza*, which can follow grief and mourning due to a loss or separation.

A second key element of the belief system underlying *curanderismo* is that illness is "God's will" or the manifestation of a saint's displeasure or anger. A closely related belief is that illness can be and is cured by God and that certain people (i.e., *curanderas*) can and do heal in God's name. Treatments for illnesses seen as essentially spiritual in their nature and cause include the lighting of candles, doing penance, and the offering of prayers to God or patron saints (Fishman et al., 1993; Gonzalez-Swafford & Gutierrez, 1983; Marsh & Hentges, 1988).

Another central feature of the belief system is that illness may be inflicted on its victim by unnatural or mystical forces, both intentionally and unintentionally. For example, *mal puesto* is believed to be an evil illness intentionally inflicted on its victim by the hex of a *bruja* (witch) or some other person skilled in witchcraft. The infliction of this illness is thought to be prompted by jealousy. Symptoms include sudden attacks of screaming, crying, or singing, convulsions, and uncontrolled urination; treatments involve massage, herbs, prayer, and making crosses on the arms with a mixture of olive oil and chili powder (Fishman et al., 1993).

Just as balance and harmony are important in the emotional, spiritual, and social realms, they are also critical in the physical realm. Imbalance in the physical realm, as in the other realms, can cause illness, and one's health depends on maintaining a proper balance between "hot" and "cold" substances in the body. *Hot* illnesses can be caused by excessive consumption of hot foods. Gonzalez-Swafford and Gutierrez (1983) offer the following description of hot foods, illnesses, and treatments:

> Hot foods are not necessarily spicy or hot in their temperature, but are considered hot solely because of their effects on the body. Some foods considered to be hot are aromatic beverages, chili, expensive meats (beef, water

fowl, mutton, and fish), and wheat products. Examples of illness caused by eating an excess of hot foods include stomach ulcers, *empacho* (indigestion, infection), and *colico* (nausea and vomiting, abdominal cramps). Hot illnesses are treated by ridding the body of excess heat, thus restoring equilibrium. Usually, this is done through the use of cooling herbs brewed as tea, enemas which are thought to remove heat, or by a change in diet to include more foods considered cold. (p. 31)

Conversely, *cold* illnesses are believed to be caused by overexposure to cold weather or excessive consumption of cold foods, and the treatment entails the ingestion of hot foods, herbs, and beverages.

Who Uses Curanderismo and Why

Older Mexican Americans are more likely to have stronger religious and superstitious beliefs than are the younger population (Gonzalez-Swafford & Gutierrez, 1983). Because of superstition and emphasis on the religious and supernatural in *curanderismo,* one might speculate, then, that practice of *curanderismo* is more common among the older generations of Mexican Americans than among the younger generations. Unfortunately, few data are available on the age of users in the literature on *curanderismo.* One exception is the study of *curanderismo* utilization among Mexican Americans in the southwestern United States, conducted by Higginbotham, Trevino, and Ray (1990). These researchers reported no significant age difference between users and nonusers of *curanderismo* as well as no significant differences in marital status, family size, poverty status, insured status, or regular source of conventional health care.

This study also reports that only 4.2% of the respondents reported consulting a *curandera, herbalista,* or other folk medicine practitioner in the past 12 months. Those who did were slightly more likely to be male, less well educated, and foreign born than those who did not. The sample for this survey included 3,623 adult Mexican Americans; 58% were male and 42% were female (Higginbotham et al., 1990). The fact that females were somewhat underrepresented in the survey is significant because other researchers (Gonzalez-Swafford & Gutierrez, 1983) report that women are the primary caregivers and health care decision makers in the Mexican American community. Other factors that may influence the rates of reported use are the language in which the interview is conducted and the precise manner in which interview questions are translated, worded, or posed. Higginbotham et al. (1990), for example, found that being interviewed in Spanish was highly predictive of *curandera* utilization.

In a separate study of *curandera* utilization in Laredo, Texas, all interviews were conducted in Spanish by local residents who underwent a week's training in interviewing techniques (McKee, 1992). Researchers in this study found that interviewers who used the terms *curandera* or *curanderismo* reported little or no utilization of *curanderas* by the subjects interviewed. However, when the question was rephrased by one interviewer, the responses were markedly different. Rather than asking respondents "Do you use a *curandera* for health care?" this particular interviewer phrased the question in Spanish in the following manner: "When someone in your family is ill with *susto* or *empacho* . . . or something like that, do you know how to cure him or her, or do you know someone who does?" (McKee, 1992, p. 361). When phrased in this way, almost all of the survey respondents answered this question affirmatively and proceeded to describe their experiences with several folk illnesses and *curanderismo* treatments and remedies. McKee (1992) provides this explanation:

> Clearly, even in Laredo's impoverished barrios, people are well aware of the opprobrium attached to curanderismo, especially when it is clearly identified by the traditional lexical label. They are embarrassed to admit that they resort to it when asked directly, but readily describe their use of the system when the interviewer, a member of their own community, both assumes that they use it and refrains from labeling." (p. 361)

Results from another study of *curanderismo* utilization in Lubbock, Texas, appear to reinforce this idea. Marsh and Hentges (1988) found that only 7% of the participants in their study responded affirmatively when asked if they had seen a *curandera*. However, when asked to describe their experiences with specific illnesses and treatments, more than half of the respondents reported using conventional medical treatments *and* traditional folk remedies associated with *curanderismo*. These different findings highlight the need for researchers to (1) distinguish between the actual consulting of a *curandera* and the use of traditional *curanderismo* remedies, (2) emphasize the importance of conducting interviews in Spanish, and (3) be sensitive to and familiar with community norms and beliefs.

As Marsh and Hentges (1988) note, debate continues over whether folk remedies are used primarily for cultural or economic reasons. They also note that the results of their study indicate that the practice of *curanderismo* does not appear to be limited to any one socioeconomic or demographic segment of the Mexican American population studied. Their study found no significant differences between users and nonusers of *curanderismo* remedies in terms of economic status, education, family size, or primary language. These findings seem to argue against policymakers who attribute the myriad of health care problems suffered by poorly educated, poverty-level Mexican Americans to their adherence to *curanderismo*, because better educated and higher-income Mexican Americans also use *curanderismo* remedies.

Puerto Ricans and Espiritismo, *Cubans and* Santeria

Gomez and Gomez (1985) note both similarities and differences among the healing beliefs and practices of Mexican Americans, Puerto Ricans, and Cuban Americans. Similarities include the significant influence on all three of Catholicism and traditional Spanish medicine. The strong religious influence on health beliefs among Mexican Americans was discussed above. Similar religious beliefs are held by non-Mexican Hispanic Americans. In one study of non-Mexican Hispanic Americans, 78% of the patients reported believing that their diabetes was the result of "God's will" (Zaldivar & Smolowitz, 1994). Seventeen percent of the patients in this study also reported using herbal remedies to treat their diabetes. Thirty-five percent of the patients were born in Puerto Rico, and 8% were born in Cuba.

Mexican American *curanderismo* differs from the traditional Puerto Rican healing system, known as *espiritismo* (see more on this practice in chapter 11), and the traditional Cuban healing system, known as *santeria*, in that it has a much stronger Native American influence. In contrast, Puerto Rican *espiritismo* and Cuban *santeria* are influenced more by African customs because of the relatively larger slave populations on these islands. Traditional Puerto Rican healers, know as *espiritistas*, are believed to be able to communicate with the spirit world in order to heal illnesses and solve other problems. Traditional Cuban healers, known as *santeros*, act as both diagnosticians and healers. Their healing rituals often entail seances and animal sacrifices (Gomez & Gomez, 1985).

NATIVE AMERICANS

Although Native Americans comprise less than 1% of the total population of the United States, their culture and customs have long been a focus of study. The Native American population is diverse and heterogeneous, with approximately 500 federally recognized tribes and an additional estimated 100 tribes that are not recognized by the federal government (Kramer, 1992). Traditional Native American medical systems vary from tribe to tribe, but most share a set of common beliefs, rituals, and practices. The focus of the following discussion is on those beliefs and practices that are shared by many different Native American tribes.

Beliefs/Belief Systems

Disease or illness in the Native American tradition is commonly believed to be caused by "some disharmony in the cosmic order, as well as hexing, breaking a taboo, fright, or soul loss" (Achterberg, 1988, p. 74). The concept of disease and illness in the Native American tradition differs substantially from that of Western/Anglo-American biomedicine. In contrast to conventional biomedicine, Kramer (1992) describes the traditional Native American system of healing as "holistic and wellness oriented. It focuses on behaviors and life-styles through which harmony can be achieved in the physical, spiritual, and personal aspects of one's roles in the family, community, and environment" (p. 281). Common rituals and treatments in the Native American tradition are sweating and purging, herbal remedies (see Table 9.1), and shamanic healing.

Sweating and purging are used to purify and strengthen the body and the spirit. Although it is believed that the treatment is seldom employed today, herbal preparations such as "black drink," used by many southeastern tribes, were often used in the past to induce vomiting, thus purging impurities from the body (Hudson, 1979). Sweating is still widely practiced today, often in small conical structures known as "sweat lodges," where hot rocks are doused with water to produce steam. Sweating is used as a form of preventive medicine as well as a form of healing (McGaa, 1990). In the Lakota community, one of several branches in the Sioux tribe, the sweat lodge ceremony sometimes lasts several hours. It is used as a means of arriving at major decisions or dealing with difficult problems or situations and as a means of purification on a monthly basis by the tribe's men, as "a kind of parallel to women's monthly menses" (National Institutes of Health, 1994, p. 97).

Virtually all Native American tribes are believed to use or have used some forms of herbal remedies in their healing rituals and practices. *The Handbook of Northeastern Indian Medicinal Plants* (Duke, 1986) lists several of these remedies, a number of which are described in Table 9.1.

Native American "holy people," or shamans, use very naturalistic and personalistic healing practices. Shamanism is believed to still be widely practiced in several Native American tribes. The shamanic practices of the Lakota Sioux and the Dineh, or Navajo, tribes are among the better-documented practices and are believed to be illustrative of the different and varied shamanistic practices of many Native American tribes (National Institutes of Health, 1994).

In the Lakota tribes, medicine and religion are seen as inseparable, as are the body and spirit. Their healing practices and ceremonies are led by specialists, usually referred to as medicine women or men, and are shamanistic in nature (Hulkrantz, 1985). Medicine women and men are believed to discover their calling through dreams and visions. In the case of some, this calling is sought out in a "vision quest." In other cases, the calling is believed to be unsought, appearing in lucid dreams or during serious illness. In either case medicine women or men must go through extensive training and are expected to successfully demonstrate their skills publicly to the tribe before beginning practice. The medicine wheel, or sacred hoop, is an

TABLE 9.1   Native American Herbal Remedies

Herb	Properties
Sweetflag or calamus	Many tribes believed that the root of this plant had mystical powers; others considered it to be a panacea. It is used to treat a wide spectrum of problems, including flatulence, bowel problems, colds, coughs, sore throats, headaches, colic, cholera, spasms, suppressed menses, and yellowish urine.
Coneflower (*echinacea*)	Echinacea, a purple coneflower, is used to increase resistance to infection, bad coughs, fever, dyspepsia, insect bites, venereal disease, and blood disease.
Lobelia	The leaves of lobelia are sometimes brewed as a tea and used to treat colds, croup, nosebleeds, fever, headaches, rheumatism, and syphilis. They contain the chemical lobeline sulfate, which is used in antitobacco therapy. Lobelia is also used as an antiasthmatic, an expectorant, and treatment for bronchitis and tuberculosis.
Bloodroot	This plant is used as a pain reliever and sedative and to treat chronic bronchitis, diphtheria, sore throats, deafness, dyspepsia, and uterine and other cancers. It is a very poisonous plant, and in Appalachia it is used as a charm to ward off evil spirits.
Mayapple	This plant is used to treat venereal warts and as a treatment for tumors. It is also used to treat snakebite and as an insecticide for potato bugs.
White willow	The leaves and bark of this tree, which contain the same acid used to make aspirin, are used to treat calluses, corns, warts, tumors, and cancers. Tea made from the leaves and bark is also used to reduce fevers.
Wild cherry	The bark of this tree is used to treat colds, coughs, sore throats, tuberculosis, sores and wounds, diarrhea, and stomach cramps.

Source: Duke (1986).

elaborate ceremony led by the medicine women and men of the Lakota tribe. The wheel, or hoop, is divided into four quadrants, each possessing a distinct character or power. The four quadrants are separated into two roads, a red one for happiness and a black one for sorrow. The ceremony, which involves prayers to tribal ancestors, is believed to be healing for all those who participate in it (Black Elk & Lyon, 1990; McGaa, 1990).

The Dineh, or Navajo, are concentrated in the southwestern United States, and are the largest Native American tribe in North America today. Dineh/Navajo healers fall into two categories—singers and diagnosticians. A central belief in the Navajo tradition is that balance, harmony, happiness, and connection to community are essential to one's health. In keeping with this belief, singing ceremonies are attended by large numbers of the community. Presence at the ceremony is believed to be healing for all who attend, even though it is generally focused on healing a particular individual. Singers, who lead the tribe in the ceremony, are very knowledgeable about herbal remedies, which also are used in the ceremonies. Singers are not shamans and are not believed to be called to their practice, as are the diagnosticians. Some of the chants performed by the singers during the ceremony are of epic length and can take years to learn (National Institutes of Health, 1994).

As noted, diagnosticians are believed to be called to their practices, usually though some unusual experience. Some diagnoses are performed in a deep trance by "hand tremblers" or "star gazers." Hand tremblers go into a deep trance, during which they pass their trembling hands over the body of the patient. When their hands reach the location on the patients where the illness is located, their hands suddenly cease trembling, and the diagnosis is completed. Star gazers, as the name indicates, read the stars while in a deep trance. It is believed that information regarding illness can be found in the stars and that star gazers possess a special ability to read this information from the stars while in a trance and then make a diagnosis. Listeners are a third type of diagnostician, but unlike the hand tremblers and star gazers they do not perform their diagnoses in a trance. Rather, they listen to what patients have to say and make a diagnosis based on that information. The diagnosis is usually traced to some deep cause and is reported in terms of harmony and disharmony (Topper, 1987).

Who Uses Traditional Native American Medicine and Why

It is believed that shamanism is still widely practiced in several Native American tribes today. For example, traditional healing practices among the Lakota and Navajo tribes, which were described above, are believed to be relatively well maintained and documented. Information on the current use of traditional healing methods among other Native American tribes is more limited. The authors of the 1994 Report to the NIH on Alternative Medicine state that "among Native American Indians living today there are many stories about seemingly impossible cures that have been wrought by holy people. However, the information on what was done is closely guarded and not readily rendered to non-Native American investigators" (p. 99).

Other researchers have made similar comments on the lack of data available in this area, particularly the extremely limited data on the health care of urban Native Americans (Kramer, 1992). Kramer also notes that cultural and economic barriers prevent many urban Native Americans, particularly the elderly, from accessing conventional medical care.

Although these findings are useful in assessing the extent of use of non-Native American health services (i.e., biomedicine) by Native Americans, they tell us little or nothing about the extent to which traditional Native American health practices are still being used by different tribes. One could speculate that usage rates of biomedicine by Native Americans might be relatively low because usage rates of traditional Native American remedies might be relatively high. Respecting Native American desires for privacy of their religious healing ceremonies, we may never know the extent to which Native American healing practices are still in use among the many different tribes.

ASIAN AMERICANS

The majority of Asian Americans may be of East Asian origin (which focuses on Chinese medicine), but there is also a growing number of South Asians who may be using Ayurveda or Unani. The following discussion focuses on East Asia and on Chinese medicine, which is rooted in Chinese culture. Variations have spread throughout other Asian countries, particularly Japan, Korea, and Vietnam. This section begins with a discussion of traditional Chinese healing beliefs and practices and continues with a discussion of some of the variations on the Chinese system adopted by other Asian populations.

Beliefs/Belief Systems

Traditional Chinese medicine developed alongside Chinese culture from its shamanic, tribal origins in the pre-Christian era. Traditional Chinese medicine is a healing system in which disease "represents a lack of harmony with the natural order; treatment is aimed at re-establishing a complex philosophical balance of mind, body and spirit" (Achterberg, 1988, p. 74). A key feature of traditional Chinese medicine is the concept of *qi* (pronounced *chee*) or vital energy. Disturbances or disharmonies in one's vital energy can lead to illness. The yin and yang harmony is one form of such vital energy. The concept of yin and yang stems from an ancient Chinese belief that

> the universe developed from two complementary opposites, "yin" (ngam) the female, and "yang" (yeuhng) the male. . . . Originally conceived as equal and complementary, the elements soon developed a hierarchic relationship juxtaposing the yang over the yin. Yin began to manifest all that was evil, negative and weak. In contrast, yang stood for all that was good, positive and strong. (Mo, 1992, p. 261)

Imbalances in the yin and yang can cause illness, and "can manifest within the functions of internal organs in the generation of metabolic energy, can propagate along energetically active channels represented on the body as the acupuncture meridians, and can undergo transformations of expression according to the system of 'five phases'" (National Institutes of Health, 1994, p. 71).

These five phases are phases of energy symbolized by the five elements of fire, earth, metal, water, and wood. Treatment in traditional Chinese medicine is aimed at restoring one's vital energy and returning harmony to the yin and yang. Traditional Chinese treatments include acupuncture, acupressure, moxibustion, cupping, *qigong,* and herbal medicine.

Acupuncture involves stimulating specific points in the body by puncturing the skin at these points with a needle. In traditional Chinese medicine it is used to regulate or correct imbalances in the flow of *qi* and to restore health. Acupuncture has received much attention from Western medical practitioners because of its demonstrated pain-relieving abilities, particularly its ability to cause surgical analgesia by releasing pain-inhibiting endorphines in the body. Acupuncture is also one of the most thoroughly researched and scrutinized alternative therapies. Research has offered compelling evidence for the efficacy of acupuncture, specifically as a treatment for conditions such as osteoarthritis, chemotherapy-induced nausea, asthma, back pain, painful menstrual cycles, bladder instability, and migraine headaches.

Acupressure also entails locating specific energy points and channels in the body. Rather than puncturing the skin with needles, as in acupuncture, the acupressure therapist applies pressure to these points in the body with his or her hand and fingertips. Moxibustion and cupping involve the same principle of locating specific energy points and channels in the body. Believed to have preceded the use of needles in acupuncture, moxibustion entails the burning of *Artemisia vulgaris* (a member of the daisy family) to heat specific energy points and channels in the body to regulate or correct the flow of *qi,* thus restoring or maintaining health. Cupping uses a vacuum, created by warming air in glass or bamboo jars, to apply suction on specific energy points and channels in the body. It is used to treat a variety of conditions, including sprains, arthritis, and bronchitis. *Qigong* entails breathing, movement, and meditation exercises, which are believed to cleanse, strengthen, and restore one's vital energy channels. It has been used to stimulate the immune system and as a form of self-help among cancer patients.

Traditional Chinese herbal medicine involves a very complex system of practices and preparations using thousands of different herbs (see Table 9.2). Several traditional Chinese herbal remedies are described in Table 9.2. Moreover, the herbal medicines used throughout other Asian countries

TABLE 9.2   Better Known Asian American Herbal Remedies

Ginseng root (*ren shen*):	Ginseng root has been used in China for centuries as a treatment for a variety of ailments. In modern times ginseng has been reported to have numerous physiological effects, including antistress capabilities, histamine response effects, delay of the effects of aging, modulations of immune functions, cardiac performance effects, and alteration of circadian rhythms by modifying neurotransmitters.
Cinnabar root (*dan shen*):	Cinnabar root has been shown to improve symptoms of patients suffering from coronary artery disease in at least two different clinical studies, each involving about 300 patients. The root works by causing dilation of the coronary arteries, thus allowing the blood to flow through more easily.
Licorice root (*gan cao*):	Licorice root preparations have been used to effectively treat tuberculosis in several large clinical studies with patients unresponsive to standard conventional treatments for the disease. It is also reported to have an effectiveness rate of about 90% in treating ulcer patients.
Chinese foxglove root (*sheng di huang*):	Studies using Chinese foxglove root preparations have shown that it improves the symptoms in rheumatoid patients, including a reduction in joint pain and swelling. Another study showed that preparations using this herb in combination with the Chinese herb (*gen cao*) are effective in treating hepatitis patients, including reduced liver and spleen size and improved liver functions.
Garlic bulb (*da suan*):	Garlic bulb preparations have demonstrated effectiveness in treating amebic dysentery. In addition, when used in combination with Chinese leek seeds, it has been shown to be effective against bacteria that are resistant to penicillin and other antibiotics.

Source: NIH (1994).

vary considerably. In Japan, for example, traditional herbal medicine, known as *kampo*, is derived from traditional Chinese medicine but includes remedies and practices indigenous to Japan. It is reported that 42.7% of Japan's Western-trained medical practitioners currently prescribe *kampo* medicines, which are covered by Japan's national health insurance policy. Traditional Korean, Vietnamese, and Mien medicine are also derived from traditional Chinese medicine but include their own unique sets of practices and remedies using herbs indigenous to their regions (Chin, 1992; Gilman, Justice, Saepharn, & Charles, 1992).

Who Uses Traditional Asian Medicine and Why

The Chinese comprise the largest segment of the Asian population in the United States, with the largest concentrations found in California, New York, Hawaii, Texas, New Jersey, Massachusetts, Illinois, and Washington (in descending order). Despite this large number, the available literature on how extensively traditional Chinese medicine is practiced among Chinese Americans today is somewhat limited. Gould-Martin and Ngin (1981) identify four categories of Chinese American households: the single sojourner, the old immigrant couple, the new immigrant family, and the acculturated suburban family (Mo, 1992). Factors such as poverty, language barriers, and residence in Chinatowns where Chinese culture still prevails are believed to inhibit the first three household types from seeking the services of Western biomedical providers. On the basis of these factors, one might speculate that these same household types are more likely to use traditional shamanistic and herbal Chinese remedies.

Some researchers have suggested that other non-Chinese Asian Americans, particularly the elderly among these populations, are more likely to rely extensively on traditional remedies for similar economic, language, and cultural reasons (Chin, 1992; Gilman et al., 1992; U.S. Department of Health and Human Services, 1995). Chin (1992) notes, for example, that traditional Korean herbal medicine, known as *hanyak,* is the healing system preferred by older Korean Americans. In a case study of one Korean American family's attempts to deal with their son's mental illness, Chin reports that the patient's father, an elderly Korean American, relied extensively on traditional Korean herbal remedies. In addition, the father even returned to Korea to consult with a *mansin,* or shaman, who advised him to find a more appropriate space for the reburial of the family's ancestors. Chin explains: "In Korean society, when divination is used to diagnose sources of mental or chronic illness, it is not uncommon to blame supernatural beings, mainly dead ancestors, or other gods or demons" (p. 307).

CONCLUSION

Scientific research findings show that social and cultural aspects play a large part in the choice to rely on alternative therapies. Users are motivated by particular concepts of disease and illness, strong religious influence on health beliefs, and the notion that using alternative modalities can improve functioning. For each of the ethnic minority population groups discussed in this chapter, the inseparability of the mind, body, and spirit and the intertwining of medicine and religion are critical both to the broad definition of healing and to shamanic practice.

A combination of factors encourages the persistence of ethnomedicine. Rootwork, *curanderismo*, traditional Native American and Chinese medicine, and herbalism are healing systems that focus on the link between maintaining balance and harmony with the natural order and improving functioning in the physical, emotional, spiritual, and social realms.

The social and cultural aspects discussed here are important in helping practitioners understand what contributes to the constellation of nontraditional therapies, as well as the economic and noneconomic factors that continue to inhibit the use of Western biomedicine. The orientation toward holistic health and wellness and a focus on achieving harmony through behaviors and lifestyles will ensure alternative medicine's advance in health care for many people in the United States, including the cultural groups mentioned above.

10

Building Medical Systems at the Household Level

Clarissa T. Kimber

It's supposed to be a professional secret, but I'll tell you anyway.
We doctors do nothing. We only help and encourage the doctor within.
—Dr. Albert Schweitzer

Although it is common to speak in terms of biomedical systems or alternative medical systems when investigating health care delivery (Chu, 1993; Laguerre, 1987), it is more realistic to conceive of the medical situation within a society as a compilation of many individual household medical systems that are constantly being formulated and reformulated over time. The medical situation is generally dynamic, characterized by innovation and sometimes by abandonment of ideas, techniques, dyadic relations, and materia medica—the various drugs and herbal, zoological, and mineral items used as medicines. More than ever before, varieties of Western biomedicine, as well as alternatives for healing and health maintenance, are being made available for selection and use by people around the world. We can conceptualize the totality of these individual household systems, together with the options and capabilities in the society, as the *potential ethnomedical system*.

This potential ethnomedical system is an attribute of societies that has become quite fluid today. It is composed of the regional variant of the Western biomedical system (Dunn, 1976); the scholarly or folk-traditional medical systems of different groups in society such as Chinese, Ayurvedic, or Kenyan (Basham, 1976; Good, 1977; Porkert, 1990); the "inherited" home remedies of the household (Curtin, 1947; Kimber, 1973); and advice from the media, or popular medicine. What these building blocks—the household medical systems—are like, how they are constructed, and the implications for their use in developing alternative medical systems is the focus of this chapter. The first part of the chapter provides a conceptual framework by discussing household medical systems in terms of dyadic client/practitioner relationships. The framework is then illustrated with examples from people of German background in the Texas hill country.

A question can be asked as to why the focus is on the household medical system instead of on a family medical system. There are two good reasons for focusing on the household. First, as families expand from one generation to the next in modern American society, the location of a nuclear family in a separate domicile is the norm. This is a newer development with some ethnic groups, but among such groups as the German Americans of the Texas hill country and even the Mexican American families along the border, the young people set up separate households and may, in fact, migrate for new economic opportunities away from the near vicinity of the original home. Families may thus be composed of numerous households, each one of which can become the locus of innovation and change. Exchanges between the nearby households of the same extended families tend to be greater than with households outside the family unit.

Second, in American health studies since the 1970s the unit of statistical data gathering was the household. Much methodological material supported the household interview component, and several reports on household interviews and instruments are available (Bonham & Corder, 1981; Cohen & Kalsbeek, 1981). The fact that the federal government settled on using the household as the primary data gathering unit and that data are available in these units, suggests that, when looking at alternative strategies in health care provision, the household unit is appropriate for facilitating comparisons. It provides a way to think about how the health care system really operates in this and other countries. By understanding what goes into it and how it is constructed and functions interpersonally, innovators in the health care field may be able to shortcut the time for acceptance of innovations and facilitate procedures for disseminating medical and health information to the public.

THE HOUSEHOLD MEDICAL SYSTEM

Each household in contemporary American society possesses a rich repository of health beliefs and practices. Ethnic origins and persuasions influence the content of the household beliefs and practices. Except for Native Americans, most Americans are products of migration. The lore carried is both like and unlike that from the home country abroad or the regional center of origin within the United States. Through culture loss, borrowing, and innovation, households engage in a number of alternative practices taken from different medical systems in constructing their particular medical system. The household medical system (HMS) evolves through time with the experience of the household members and are thus empirical systems. Households consider elements or options in strategy; have inherited medical lore from their family backgrounds, as well as how to think about maintaining health; and are influenced by the propositions of the media. All are meshed in the health services context of the locality, with some individuals in the household eligible for Medicare or the insurance programs provided by health plans at work as well as other national care programs.

When illness is recognized, a sequence of diagnostics and therapeutics is put into practice, using a variety of practitioners at each referral step. Households resemble each other in their medical systems as they share socioeconomic, ethnic, and religious characteristics. The ethnomedical system is learned as part of the society's culture. When a medical practitioner from one tradition attempts to serve a client from another culture, dissonance (lack of congruence) may cause poor communication and lead to a disappointed client and a frustrated practitioner (Kleinman, 1980; Trotter & Chavira, 1981). In such cases a traditional practitioner may be more acceptable. A frequent explanation for using a *curandera* in south Texas or a *sage femme* in Martinique is that "we can talk to each other" (Kimber, 1972, 1985). The ill persons pass along a referral system until their needs are met or they cease to expect help.

As the HMS matures, selectivity of treatment sources and the network of referrals become routine. They frequently become embedded in the women's networks that act as pathways of information about health behavior (Hassenger, 1992). They constitute part of the networks of the society that is being continuously socially reproduced in an ongoing process (Soja, 1985). The HMSs in their interaction and functioning thereby construct the structure of the ethnomedical system of that society. Through experience and habit, the exploration of alternatives to the individual household system as it is worked out becomes less and less over time. It takes some trauma or excitement in curing strategies to redirect a well-established set of health-seeking behaviors in the household.

Experiences with illness that groups have over time yield a formal body of knowledge that is codified as their medical theory of illness. These same groups will have classifications of and names for illnesses that are considered likely or possible. This is the group's medical taxonomy (Kay, 1977). Both the theory and the taxonomy are modified through time by locally initiated change and by borrowing. Where multiple medical systems exist and have persisted side by side, as in the United States, borrowing is accelerated.

The role of educational institutions, including the media, cannot be overlooked, and these can overpower the medical lore transmitted between generations. Where the taxonomies of the practitioner differ from that of the client, problems may arise.

Until recently, physicians in the United States derived their beliefs and value systems from mainstream beliefs that came from northwestern Europe. More recently, physicians have been coming from other ethnic groups, but the policies of organized medical groups have been set by the older physician group; hence, public policy in health care has been formulated in a culturally selective manner. Persons from other ethnic backgrounds feel alienated by biomedical practices and attitudes and turn to more culturally sensitive practitioners for medical treatment or opt for self-medication.

Households interact directly with a few other households with respect to their medical systems. But people are also indirectly related to others through their households, and they connect in a vast network web. Typically, members of the same family, especially households of daughters, maintain close relations with the mother's household. Near neighbors exchange information more frequently than those more spatially distant if not related by marriage. Thus, direct and indirect relations are set up between and among households. In contrast, a few households are really isolated, but they are rare. The *actual ethnomedical system* is therefore a web composed of the numerous HMSs as constructed by the households. The web of relationships is thus composed of and tied to intimately related and more indirectly related households in the society. The several HMSs involve health education practices, health and sanitation controls, risk assessment, prevention techniques, diagnosis, therapy, and rehabilitation (Dunn, 1976). This actual ethnomedical system is set in a context of locally specific public health services addressed by different political entities at different levels, such as the mosquito abatement district, the municipal water supply, and the national health system—all derived, for the most part, from the value and belief systems of the cosmopolitan medical system (Pescosolido, 1986).

DYADIC RELATIONS WITHIN AN HMS

When a client visits one of the available practitioners, a dyadic relationship is set up (Figure 10.1). The relationship may be active on the part of the client (i.e., he or she takes the initiative and manages the interview or delivers information), but more often, especially when biomedical practitioners are involved, the client is passive and the direction of information as well as power flow is from the practitioner to the patient. In traditional

P → C	**Practitioner assumes responsibility, i.e., the active role; client is passive**
P ← C	**Client assumes responsibility, i.e., active role; practitioner is passive.**
P ↔ C	**Practitioner and client exchange information, both active.**
P ↔ P	**Practitioners exchange information, both active.**
C ↔ C	**Clients exchange information, both active.**
M ↔ C	**Media transmits information, client selects information; both active.**

FIGURE 10.1   Responsibility for transfer of medical information within a dyadic system. Typically, the transfer of knowledge goes from a high-status person to one of lower status. Not all possible dyadic relations are shown in the diagram. The model of the practitioner-client dyad was developed by Lannie (1982, p. 301) from the Hayes-Bautista (1978)-model of the differences between perception of clients and practitioners.

medicine, especially folk medicine, the relationship may be and usually is two-way. The exchange is among equals in beliefs, if not in status. Frequently, interviews are conducted on the living room sofa with the two seated side by side in the home of the folk curer, especially if they are of the same sex. This equality of power characteristically makes clients more comfortable, and they tend to stay in or buy into the system.

When medical practitioners from the same medical tradition converse together, there is usually a sense of mutual respect and some real sharing of information. In this instance the dyadic relationship is mutually active, diagrammed in Figure 10.1 as power and information flow in both directions. When the practitioners are from two different medical traditions, there is less sharing, and commonly less respect is given to the traditional practitioner by the biomedical practitioner. The dyadic relation is unequal, with one dominant or more active than the other. When two potential clients are together, they usually can and do exchange information. One may be active on one occasion, and on a different occasion the other person may be the donor. Older persons tend to dominate younger ones, as between generations in families.

The client satisfies health practitioner needs with numerous dyadic relations, some active, some passive. For different conditions or states, the client will select a different practitioner or health care provider. This suggests that the multiple roles may satisfy different needs in the same person and may account for the apparent incongruity of mixing significant persons as practitioners from different backgrounds even when considering the same condition. Because experiences with these relationships are shared within the household, such consultative practices of members within the household constitutes part of the HMS's *health care network*. The other part of the network is the lay-person connections that make possible the exchange of information and medicines between households by non-practitioners. Frequently thought of as gossip about health, these discussions nonetheless are the vehicle for the exchange of much new as well as traditional or old medical expertise. These networks, which can be thought of as part of the *ethnomedical infrastructure*, exist in societies whose political entities provide either many or few of the health-related services available to the persons in those societies.

The dyadic relation between the practitioner and the individual client will vary as the value system of the pair coincide, partially coincide, or are at cross-purposes. Congruence or conflict between the practitioner and his or her clients depends on the degree of shared beliefs and practices between them. Congruence is acquired through shared early learning experiences and by extended contact of the two persons of the dyad. Conflict occurs when the treatments suggested run contrary to the implications of the belief or value system or the previously acquired understanding of the "proper" treatment. The client may temporarily suspend previously held beliefs or ideas out of respect for the practitioner. The experience of success in such a situation may lead the client to revise previously held beliefs, or it may be treated as an exceptional experience. If there is a lack of dissonance between the two members of the dyad, treatment is facilitated. The responsibility for developing the climate belongs to the practitioner, although it is often not so conceived. This may lead to much ineffectiveness on the part of the practitioner, particularly in ethnic neighborhoods or among socioeconomically deprived segments of the population (Kleinman, 1980; Merchant, 1996; Quesada & Heller, 1977). Failed opportunities may lead to further alienation of the clients.

The client may be seeing several practitioners for different conditions or as a means of reinforcement of treatment for the same condition. This assumption of responsibility may be the only active part of the client in his or her own treatment, or there may be a more active role with one practitioner than with another. Along the Texas–Mexico border a client may go to a physician for help, visit a traditional practitioner, and discuss the condition with a pharmacist (Kimber, 1972). Dyck (1995) reports that using both traditional and biomedical strategies did not appear to cause conflict for immigrant women in Vancouver. Where possible, it is desirable to bring into collaboration the several practitioners the client may be consulting. If the perceived status is very different among practitioners, much skill has to be used in the consultative interaction. As the different practitioners and the client share medical taxonomies, ideas of illness causation, and appropriate therapies, collaboration can be facilitated.

Recognizing the complexity of the dyadic relations one person is involved in, it becomes abundantly clear that, when the several members of the household discuss and act out their collective dyadic relations in the HMS, there will be similarities in dyadic relations with some practitioners. These, then, can be considered the stable dyadic relationships of the HMS. If there are significant differences between members of the household in the nature of the dyadic relation with another practitioner, this source of medical service is debated and may not remain an integral part of the HMS. The individual HMS may be more or less dynamic as the number of debated dyads declines or increases.

HMSs IN THE HILL COUNTRY OF TEXAS

In 1980, Donna Lannie and the author began a study of the different parts of the ethnomedical system of the population of Gillespie County, Texas. This county had a dominant population of 19th-century German extraction; a group of persons directly descended from old-stock White Americans from Virginia, Tennessee, and Kentucky; and Mexican Americans. Although there were some Blacks and other ethnic groups, these three were the most populous. The people of German extraction were the largest group by far, and after some initial surveys the study was redirected to examine the ethnomedical system of the people of German descent.

Open-ended interviews of adult men and women, guided by a schedule of questions, were the major source of information, although a larger group of people was surveyed by the use of the same schedule in focus-group meetings with Lannie, which provided some of the statistical data collected in the study. These interviews were conducted in the house occupied by the interviewees, and information about family members and nonfamily members living there was included. Historical information was derived from the in-depth interviews and from newspapers, family letters and journals, and materials in the Barker Collection, University of Texas at Austin. Only some of the findings will be presented here as they relate to the subject. Those interested in more details may consult the dissertation by Lannie (1982) that is available from University Microfilms, Michigan.

Virtually each person interviewed saw the medical practitioner, usually a physician, as the primary health care provider. However, a variety of biomedical practitioners were consulted in the course of a year in most households (Table 10.1). Further discussion brought to light a use of traditional medical practitioners, either from their own German ethnic heritage or as borrowings from the Mexican population. Included in the list of practitioners consulted by one person were "herb doctors," midwives, and bone

TABLE 10.1   Some Health Care Systems in German Texas Society

Health Care Practice	Means of Treatment	Client Responsibility
Faith healing		
Christian faith healing	Laying on of hands	Passive
Glaubensschwaermerei	by practitioner	Passive
Naturopathy		
Home remedies	Natural objects	Active
Hydropathy	Water	Passive
Traditional medicine	Natural objects	Passive
Media-influenced practices		
Patent medicines	Natural or artificial objects	Active
Herbal remedies (back-to-nature movement)	Natural objects	Active
Medical practices		
Chiropractic	Adjustments	Passive
Pharmacy	Natural or ethical drugs	Passive
Physician	Drugs or surgery	Passive

Adapted from Lannie, 1982, p. 2.

setters. Although reluctant at first to discuss witches and *hexen*, as confidence in the investigators developed, people became more open. They reported that these practitioners were used as a last resort and for certain illnesses that medical doctors could not cure. Only some families were willing to say that they consulted them today, but most conceded that the family had used them in the past.

Most households had one person within it or one they consulted who had a rich lore of home medical remedies with origins in Germany or from the Comanche Indians, with whom the ancestors, the earliest settlers, shared the environment at contact time between the 1840s and 1860s. The majority of these medicaments were plants, although some animal parts were used, as well as kerosene, axle grease, and dirt—naturopathy in the broadest sense (Lannie, 1982, pp. 111–226). Botanical materia medica were in 52% of the home remedies and zoological materia medica in 17% of medications. Mineral materia medica were in 18% and commercial preparations were 14% of the whole set. Water cures accounted for 13% and another 7% were a miscellany of types of cures. Because of the habit of combining elements in one medication, the sum of the above figures is greater than 100%. The majority of these were inherited from the experience of the group as migrants into Texas.

The early settlers from northern Germany colonized the area around Fredericksburg in the prairie woodlands of the Edwards Plateau of Texas beginning in 1831, with very large numbers coming in the 2 years 1844–1846 (Jordan, 1966, cited in Lannie, 1982, pp. 28–30). They came with doctors and pharmacists and carried with them a rich North European ethnomedical system. Upon their arrival the German immigrants were subjected to poor conditions and ill health. At first there were many deaths, and the health of the colony was severely assaulted by disease (Bracht, 1849/1931; Mantz, 1913; Tiling, 1913). Those that survived developed a German Texan medical tradition. Lannie (1982, p. 35) points out that a transplanted people, even with their health restored, needs to develop new medical traditions that incorporate some of their old traditions and the adoption of new ones. Morgan (1973) hypothesizes a migrant personality: "Migrants may be more receptive to a range of innovative situations, including moving to a new environment and acceptance of new ideas" (p. 865).

The Germans constructed their new ethnomedical system in the 19th century. Seeds and cuttings of food and medicinal plants brought from Germany were naturalized in the Texas soil and climate (Geiser, 1945). The local flora were examined for useful plants. Baron von Meuseback, founder of Fredericksburg, was an avid collector of plants and was keenly interested in their medical uses (King, 1967, pp. 15–16); Bracht (1849/1931) describes edible and medicinal plants native to Texas. One of the doctors in the early settlement, Christian Althaus, trained as a medic in the Prussian army and carried on a professional exchange with a Comanche medicine man, often healing the Indians sent him by his counterpart (Lannie, 1982, p. 306). From the Comanche, Althaus learned directly about the value of local botanicals.

Another biomedical practitioner, Herman Lehmann, captured by the Comanche and treated by a medicine man, collected a number of Indian remedies and learned about the native medicinal flora from them (Lehmann, 1927, p. 190). He compounded the medicines he dispensed from materials locally available. However, his daughters insisted that most of his medicines came directly from Germany because they were "better quality" than the American-grown plants. Thus, repeated supplies of European herbs consolidated a dependence on the old remedies. The attitude toward medical treatments was thus conservative and inclined toward the biomedical practices of the 19th century.

However, from the discussions with informants in the early 1980s about the actual herbal remedies in use, it became clear that sources for naturopathic materials in the 1980s seemed to be changing from European or locally procured or collected to California or Utah sources. A number of people made reference to the new herb store in the community, the proprietor of which had come from California. Informants also related being sensitive to information about herbs carried in tabloid newspapers and small herb pamphlets published by packaging companies.

Some clients were shoppers like Debbie Sauer (all names used here are pseudonyms), who were inclined to be skeptical of all practitioners and made a habit of sampling a variety of practitioners (Figure 10.2, Case A). A position held by the younger generation was that, although the old folks occasionally consulted a faith healer, they were modern and would have no interaction with faith healers, considering them either charlatans or irrelevant to their own needs (Case B). One woman interviewed, Mrs. Paul Lange, took the position that she could benefit from consulting a large number of practitioners, not necessarily all at the same time for the same ailment, but she would maintain a variety of "consultants" (author's term) (Case C). In this instance, she was the active one in the dyads and saw the pharmacist as giving her much the same information as the physician even though he did not know as much, but she always consulted with him because he was more likely to discuss the case with her than the physician. Some persons, like Herman Keidel, were more inclined to consult a chiropractic practitioner only (Case D). Others, like Tilly Otto, refused to consider consulting a practitioner even as a possible option (Case E) because of the lack of congruity between them as perceived by her.

The decision as to whom to consult develops as a household decision. People said such things as "we use such and such a person" or "our family doesn't pay much attention to . . ." Patterns had developed over time as to whom to consult for what. The community was small enough so that virtually all the persons knew all the health practitioners in the county, with the exception of the faith healers, who were often family members not shared with the rest of the community.

Individuals discussed their relationship with different health practitioners. Most had an uneven, dependent relationship with physicians and chiropractic practitioners but one of equality or mutual exchange with pharmacists, faith healers, and herb doctors. With *hexen* the relationship was guarded, and there was more distance. Dyadic relations thus varied according to practitioner. There was a tendency to have more affectionate respect for a doctor who had been the family physician since the informant was a child. Physicians were often consulted for advice on other biomedical specialists such as cardiologists, internists, and brain surgeons. All informants, when asked directly, said they did not mention going to alternative practitioners to their physicians. When asked why not, they answered that there was "not much point in it," "they [biomedical practitioners] aren't interested in discussing such people," or "they are antagonistic toward them."

Most people interviewed said they were interested in looking after themselves because medicines were getting more expensive and doctors

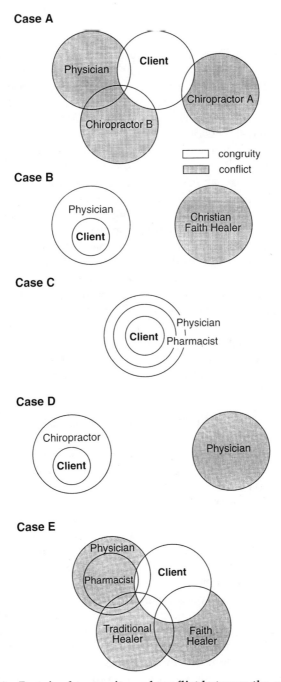

Case A

Client

Physician

Chiropractor A

Chiropractor B

☐ congruity
▨ conflict

Case B

Physician

Client

Christian
Faith Healer

Case C

Client

Physician

Pharmacist

Case D

Chiropractor

Client

Physician

Case E

Physician

Pharmacist

Client

Traditional
Healer

Faith
Healer

FIGURE 10.2   Perceived congruity and conflict between the assessments of client-self and the practitioners. Only five of the possible cases are diagrammed. From Lannie, 1982, pp. 15, 311–314.

were also expensive. There was an interest in preventive medicine, and it was clear that the wellness movement was taking hold in the county. However, most people did not have a sophisticated understanding of newer health care practices. Rural residents had a marginally stronger background in herbal preparations and more independence in decision making than the residents of the city and towns.

The study area, Gillespie County, and the study group, German Americans, are a well-knit cultural area and society. The German population is interconnected by marriage ties and by shared histories of medical experiences. Some of the older people reported that their mothers had told them not to play with the Americans, implying that the latter were inferior to themselves. This self-imposed segregation tied the Germans more tightly together and maintained the distinction of that community from the other groups in the county. Besides the internal network of associations of the various HMSs, some members of the society do seek help from practitioners outside the area. San Antonio is a large metropolitan area not far away, with a rich set of cosmopolitan medical resources associated with university complexes; so in the case of the German Americans of Gillespie County, the ethnomedical system includes some extraterritorial providers and services. The local ethnomedical system intersects with other local systems. In such a way hierarchies of medical systems are actually constructed.

SUMMARY AND CONCLUSIONS

It has been proposed that households are the basic units of an ethnomedical system of any particular society. The HMS is the setting in which decisions are initiated concerning the health of members of the household and of numerous relations with a variety of health practitioners. Early in the formation of the HMS, as an illness is identified, discussions with a variety of persons in a network identify a suitable remedy from the household lore or a specific practitioner is consulted. Individuals within the household interact with one another in consultation and decision making; and eventually, as an illness is identified, appropriate action becomes codified, even routinized. The different dyadic relations of the individual members of the household with the practitioner create a dynamic that is a part of a functioning system. The particular amount of use of home remedies, old folk traditions, traditional medical practitioners, and biomedical practitioners is unique to each HMS. Within a community the various households are linked, directly through a consultation process or indirectly via others, to make up the real or actual ethnomedical system of that society.

As elements in and parts of folk and other alternative medical systems continue to mainstream and as biomedicine attempts popularization through accessibility, the separateness of these different medical systems is becoming blurred (Albuquerque, 1979). Efforts in Nigeria, Mexico, and Ghana suggest that professional collaboration between practitioners of different medical systems in a society can help improve the level of health care for the population if they can overcome their lack of confidence in each other (World Health Organization, 1992, 1993). Where there is mutual respect through shared or acknowledged taxonomies, the collaboration will be expedited (Alvarado, 1978).

Regional health care systems in the worldwide biomedical tradition can be designed that will maximize the use of the actual ethnomedical system of the region. However, there must remain enough flexibility so that the individual household has the ability to carry out its own strategy or HMS. Health promoters and health planners can facilitate such an ability by being conscious of its presence and characteristics and be committed to working with it.

The richness of the actual ethnomedical system is often ignored or not perceived by persons interested in health care delivery. The fact that it is not capitalized on reduces the effectiveness of political measures directed toward improving health and points up the weaknesses in the delivery of medicine in the society. A healthier society can result at lower cost with the effective use of the diversities in the HMS.

11

Redefining the Healing Process: Healer–Client Relationships in Alternative Medicine

Joan D. Koss-Chioino

I said to the Almond tree
"Sister, speak to me of God"
and the Almond tree blossomed.
—St. Francis of Assisi

A focus on the therapist–patient/client relationship as central to therapeutic process originally stems from the work of Freud and his followers in psychoanalysis, who framed it in terms of transference of early childhood feelings to the analyst and countertransference or response on his or her part. More recently, in research in psychotherapy, the therapist-client relationship has been looked upon as central to therapeutic effectiveness and demonstrated to be significant for outcomes (Henry, Schact, & Strupp, 1986; Horvath & Greenberg, 1986; Luborsky, McLellan, Woody, O'Brien, & Auerbach, 1985; Marziali & Alexander, 1991; Orlinsky & Howard, 1975). Recent attention has also been given to doctor-patient relationships with regard to their impact on various aspects of patient care, such as compliance with treatment or speed of recovery from various procedures (Ayanian & Epstein, 1991; Hall, Epstein, DeCiantis, & McNeil, 1993; Hall, Roter, & Katz, 1988). Even the allied health disciplines, such as occupational therapy, concern themselves with the qualities of the therapeutic relationship because it is "the most significant element in facilitating therapy" (Lloyd & Maas, 1991, p. 111). Although each of these health care disciplines describes the ideal therapeutic relationship in somewhat different ways, there is widespread agreement on some of the basic (i.e., ideal) characteristics of the therapist/provider, such as warmth, caring, attentiveness, and credibility, and on relationship qualities such as mutual affirmation and receptivity and good communication that takes emotions into account. In one study three of the major alliance measures were shown to have convergent as well as discriminant validity as rated by both therapists and clients (Bachelor, 1991). Clients who perceive greater levels of positive characteristics of therapists improve most.

Although the literature on the therapeutic relationship is extensive, most studies and descriptions conform to a paradigm common to orthodox medical and mental health care practice and rarely consider features or patterns outside a dyadic model of relationship, the features of which are based largely on behavioral evidence. The goal of this chapter is to introduce a very different model of relating between healers and clients, one that constitutes the healing process in numerous traditional and folk practices. This model is common to healing rituals that involve spirits or gods who manifest as a crucial part of the healing act, but its parameters may be applicable to other types of healing systems. In contrast to the medical model, a therapeutic dyad is not central; instead, there is a triadic or polymorphic relationship, constituted by a client/petitioner, a healer, and one or more extraordinary beings. This is well described in an abundant anthropological literature on shamanism and traditional healing (Boddy, 1989; Koss-Chioino, 1992, 1995; Peters, 1981, among many others).

This differently structured relationship facilitates the healing process in ways distinct from those described or assumed for orthodox medical or psychological practices. First, it is not based on a paradigm in which the therapeutic encounter is between two individuals of unequal power and authority. Second, it is not oriented solely toward individuals per se but much more commonly involves a context in which individual sufferers are treated as members of a class or group. And third, the healing process depends on bringing the individual into contact with significant extraordinary aspects of his or her life world, beyond the visible world of immediate existence, such as the realm of the ancestors, the world of spirits, or the sphere of the Godhead, whether Christian, Muslim, Jewish, or Zoroastrian. I suggest that an understanding of the patterning of the healing relationship, as contrasted with the therapeutic relationship (to make a terminological distinction), can illuminate aspects of healing relationships in alternative medical practices, at the same time perhaps helping to account for some healing processes in orthodox biomedical practices that are considered different, such as hypnotherapy.

This chapter briefly reviews some of the descriptions of therapeutic relationships in psychology, psychoanalysis, biomedicine, and allied health disciplines as well as in literature that takes a cross-cultural perspective. It is not intended as an overview of the topic but focuses instead on variations and critiques of the way the model of the therapeutic relationship is typically described. The healing relationship and healing process in *Espiritismo*—a traditional cult religion in Puerto Rico found (with variations) in almost all Latin American and some Mediterranean societies—is then described (Harwood, 1977; Koss-Chioino, 1992). It is offered as an illustration of a model for conceptualizing and structuring healing relationships alternative to that prescribed for current health and mental health care practitioners.

This approach then sets up a comparison aimed at understanding the healing process in alternative medicine. The interpretation offered here is intended as a contribution to the general goal of redefining the healing process so as to more closely approximate a universal model (Koss-Chioino, 1992, 1996). However, the goal is not only to contribute to an understanding of salient aspects of the healing process that are of theoretical interest but also to fulfill a practical need, because traditional healing practices are widespread in the United States, especially among ethnic minority and immigrant communities (Koss-Chioino, 1995). To that end, the impact of the societal context of healing practices on their form and structure is also part of this analysis because traditional healing, as well as healing in general, is not just an event occurring between individuals but both reflects and reproduces a wide range of sociocultural factors.

THE THERAPEUTIC RELATIONSHIP

PSYCHOTHERAPY

As Marziali and Alexander (1991) point out, the psychodynamic and behavioral perspectives in psychotherapy differ with regard to views on the centrality of the therapeutic relationship to treatment. In the case of psychodynamic psychotherapies, the therapist role provides both the container and the agent of change when an interpretation of the therapeutic relationship is applied to explaining a client's maladaptive relationships outside therapy. However, in the case of the behavioral therapies, the therapeutic relationship serves as a context (a container) for interventions aimed to bring about change in the client. With regard to both of these psychotherapeutic modalities (and others, such as cognitive behavioral interventions), the important question is, what are essential ingredients for change? Because various types of modalities have been demonstrated to be effective, many speculations but few studies of common change processes are available. The therapeutic bond has been the most studied aspect of therapeutic process (Orlinsky, Grawe, & Parks, 1994) and ranks as the primary candidate in finding a factor common to therapeutic change in general.

Of the many formulations of the characteristics of the therapeutic relationship, Bordin's (1979) early description of three dimensions forms the structure for many subsequent measures: (1) therapist's and client's agreement on goals, (2) therapist's and client's agreement on tasks to achieve these goals, and (3) development of a bond between them. These measures phrase the relationship somewhat differently. For example, (1) the Relationship Inventory (Barrett-Lennard, 1986) examines four dimensions—positive regard, empathic understanding, unconditionality of regard, and congruence; (2) the Therapy Session Report (Orlinsky & Howard, 1975) focuses on three dimensions—mutual affirmation, mutual receptivity, and sensitive collaboration; (3) in the Penn Alliance Scales, completed by both client and therapist (Luborsky et al., 1985), two different aspects are associated with outcome—a Type I alliance, in which the client perceives the therapist as having the major responsibility, and a Type II alliance, in which the client perceives the therapy to be a collaborative process. Type II relationships are associated with more positive outcomes after 7 months of treatment.

All of these instruments are based on the same point of departure, that of the importance of a special *interpersonal* relationship and how it is perceived by each member. Measures of the therapeutic alliance are generally taken after three sessions, near the beginning of treatment (which can last for many months depending on the modality). Ratings of the client's alliance behavior are more highly predictive of outcome than are ratings of therapist behavior; the implication is that the quality of the client's relationship with the therapist is a crucial, if not the most crucial, aspect of therapeutic success. Some studies suggest that clients who exhibit extreme or abnormal interpersonal behavior have difficulty forming a working alliance with the therapist and vice versa (Kiesler & Watkins, 1989).

If we construct a comparison between therapist-patient relationships and those integral to traditional healing practices, the healer-client relationship must be observed to have a different structure and dynamic because there are three or more parties to the healing encounter. By its very nature a triadic relationship is much more complex compared to the ways the therapist-client relationship is conceptualized and enacted. With regard to bonding, for example, one can ask, with whom—healer or spiritual being? Moreover, what is the nature and quality of the bond with either one? Clearly, in comparing bonds with spirits versus bonds with healers, different relationship rules apply. How are these multifaceted relationships related to engaging a client in treatment or his or her continued attendance (most clients come only once or sporadically)? Is "complementarity" or a "mutualism" a necessary element in the healer-client relationship?

Such factors may be important only to healer apprentices or persons with chronic illnesses who have a continuous relationship with a healer. Evidence is equivocal regarding the extent to which healer and client must share beliefs; "similarity of values" may be irrelevant to the main goals of traditional healing practices (Kelly & Strupp, 1992). In Spiritist and other Hispanic healing practices, the goal of the ritual healing session is to "take off" the harmful spirit or other illness-causing beings or to cleanse the sufferer's body of the noxious material or spiritual substances causing distress, rather than to bring about cognitive change through understanding, insight, or redirected behavior patterns (Koss-Chioino, 1992).

PSYCHOANALYTIC DISCIPLINES

Although historically the therapist-patient relationship is a descendant of what is now known as the psychoanalytic schools of theory and practice, there are some basic differences between it and the analyst-analysand relationship. The intensity of the treatment and its much longer duration provide parameters somewhat different from those of psychotherapeutic alliances. The concept and process of transference is central to psychoanalytic and psychodynamic therapists. In Freud's later formulations the core of analytic work is the transference neurosis, typified by the patient's transferring aspects of early experience (particularly traumatic ones) to his or her analyst. Treatment revolves around resolution of this neurotic state reenacted within the therapeutic setting. Although this originally implied a projection from patient to therapist, more recent psychoanalytic schools focus equally on countertransference—the therapist's unconscious response to his or her patient's projections. This does not include the role of the therapist's personality in the formation of the transference, however, which is related to how the therapist is behaving toward the patient and the need to make this behavior conscious (Stein, 1973).

Analytical psychologists who follow C. G. Jung view the dynamics of transference as occurring on both sides of the therapeutic dyad; in one formulation the patient projects his or her inner healer onto the analyst. According to Jungian thought, the "wounded" patient also contains his or her opposite, the physician or healer. The same is true for the therapist, who very often is (or has been) wounded and may project his or her woundedness onto the patient, thus preventing change or healing from taking place. To promote change, in Jungian terms, a "third quantity," an archetypal image, is constellated in the unconscious that activates the patient's `inner' healer (Groesbeck, 1975, p. 131). As I have described elsewhere, this is very similar to that which occurs in spirit healing, where the "third quantity" is personified as a spirit being (Koss-Chioino, 1992).

PHYSICIAN-PATIENT RELATIONSHIP

Doctor-patient relationships are frequently described as "problematic" because of poor communication and failure of trust (Lazarus, 1988). The picture of a paternalistic, authoritarian physician and a dependent, sub-missive patient is typical to most descriptions even though discussed as undesirable in the social science literature. A key issue is that of power, whether conceptualized as power to make clinical and other decisions for a patient or as control over resources (Pappas, 1990). As Pappas (1990) aptly notes: "power cuts two ways: it both constrains and enables" (p. 200). When patients are asked about the need for egalitarianism in their dealings with doctors, they do not always agree that they want more control over their treatment (Lupton, Donaldson, & Lloyd, 1991). Patients most often advance the notion that trust is the most important component of their rela-tionship with physicians. Yet control over resources can lead to domination, as well as to exploitation in matters of health and illness. Relationship with a physician-healer can be appreciated as a two-edged sword: caring, cur-ing, and relief are the benefits of trust and authority, but the price may be domination over life decisions, disease definition, and values.

CROSS-CULTURAL PERSPECTIVES

Despite the large-scale exportation of the enterprise of psychotherapy, rel-atively little exploration of the therapeutic alliance in other cultures has taken place. Ivey (1987) indirectly questions the validity of a two-person construct in the therapeutic relationship on cultural grounds when he asserts: "It could be said that four participants may be found in the inter-view: the therapist and her or his cultural background and the client and his or her cultural background" (p. 197). He focuses on the ethical dimen-sion of the therapeutic enterprise by deconstructing the aspect of "empa-thy," which he insists requires that the therapist not only understand the client as a unique being but also understand the sociohistorical context in which that person is embedded. Being empathically understood and val-ued has been linked to reparative effects on the client's experience of and sense of self (Kohut, 1984). However, following Ivey (1987), the question is raised about how empathy is defined; moreover, the patient or client must be considered within the context of her or his lifeway, including notions about relationships with a therapist or health care provider.

In contrast to popular notions about empathic understanding as a cen-tral feature of verbal communication between therapists and clients, I suggest that empathy, as an element of the therapeutic situation, can be achieved in nonverbal, impersonal ways by facilitating and/or fostering the relationship of a client to an extraordinary being, force, or notion. This idea will be further explicated below.

These perspectives are directly applicable to ethnic minority populations in the United States, as well as to persons in other cultures. They have led to an extended discussion of whether therapists and clients should be ethnically and culturally matched and whether therapists and counselors should adopt roles alternative to the orthodox (often highly formalized), one-to-one relationship at the therapist's office (Edwards, 1988; Foulks & Pena, 1995; Sue & Sue, 1990). Thus far, however, cultural matching of therapist and client has not been demonstrated to improve outcomes in treatment (Sue, 1988). Alternative approaches to the more formalized psychotherapeutic modalities are increasingly being developed (e.g., multidimensional family therapy); but their ethnic or cultural specificity, particularly in relation to therapeutic effectiveness, has only begun to be demonstrated (Koss-Chioino & Vargas, 1992: Rogler, Malgady, Costantino, & Blumenthal, 1987). It has even been suggested that the entire enterprise of psychotherapy may be inappropriate or antagonistic for many minority group individuals, who may be reluctant to talk about their problems and/or to disclose intimate experiences to a stranger (Sue & Sue, 1990).

With regard to the doctor-patient relationship, Lazarus (1988) raises a further issue of considerable importance. She suggests that in addition to locating doctor-patient relationships within a macro-sociopolitical context, in relation to factors that structure medical systems, two other areas of study are essential: the social interaction between doctor and patient and the particular features of the institution where treatment takes place. This raises the specter of the effects of sociocultural distance on the relationship between a middle-class or elite health care provider with professional status and a lower-class patient who is a lay person in the medical system and who also may be a member of a denigrated ethnic minority group.

That social distance can inhibit therapeutic success has been accepted at face value because it can block cooperation and mutuality; at least one study (Coady, 1991) shows that therapists in poor-outcome cases of psychodynamic psychotherapy expressed significantly more communications discouraging affiliative interactions and significantly more interpretive communications that defeated affiliation with these patients. These communications were frequently interpretations about their relationship with the client. However, perhaps the basic issue that should be considered is that of power relations in terms of degrees of autonomy and dependency or, more broadly, in terms of domination over healing resources (Pappas, 1990). Doctors and many types of health care providers have greater decision-making power and control over resources than do patients as part of their institutional roles; societal relationships hinged on power differentials as additional elements of the therapeutic relationship can only exacerbate these differences.

TRADITIONAL HEALING: AN ALTERNATIVE PERSPECTIVE ON PROCESS

Having considered a diversity of perspectives that have been offered to explain salient aspects (both positive and negative) of the therapeutic relationship in psychotherapeutic and biomedical healing, this section focuses on contrasting perspectives that emerge in the study of traditional healing, some of which have been briefly described previously. To illustrate differences in healing relationships in traditional and folk healing, a session from the author's research in Puerto Rico is described.

AT A SPIRITIST SESSION IN PUERTO RICO

The room seemed crowded with rows of folding chairs filled with people who spoke very little except for occasional quiet whispers to their neighbors. Behind a long table covered with a white cloth sat five women and one man, three of whom had on white starched clothing similar to that worn by doctors or lab technicians. There was a squat crystal bowl of water in the center of the table out of which leaned one long-stemmed red rose. The mediums sitting behind the table leaned into their cupped hands or stared with seemingly unfocused eyes at those assembled in front of them.

The appointed president of this group of mediums rose from her seat in the middle of the table. She enjoined the audience to open their arms and uncross their legs. She then proceeded to open the session with a short prayer about peace and harmony and began to read from *The Bible According to Spiritism* by Allan Kardec. The participants' attentions were directed to the sacred world of God, the saints, and the spirits of persons once incarnate. Then the president signaled silence and told the audience to meditate on the spirit world. The mediums seemed to be readying themselves to "call" their spirit-guide-protectors into their bodies. (Mediums' bodies are "vessels" *[cajas]* that can be opened to receive spirit vibrations or presences; prayers and meditation are psychic means to achieve a special state in which to communicate with the spirit world.)

Once their spirit guides were present, the mediums visibly relaxed in their chairs and seemed to be heavily concentrating on trying to see events in the spirit world that involved persons in the audience. One of the mediums, a stocky woman in a white uniform, whispered something to the president. Apparently she had an experience *(una videncia)* of the spirit world. The person to whom the vision pertained was pointed out as "that young woman in the blue dress." The president beckoned to her to stand in front of the table opposite the medium. The medium then asked if she had a headache, but not "too bad," was "seeing double and had bad eyesight," and "had a tired head." Had she had been "pacing through her house without a direction"? Was she "worried about her youngest son"? At each question the woman answered, "Yes" or "Sure." The possessed medium had molded or formed this woman's pains and emotional distress within her own body, and the young woman understood that the medium was experiencing her feelings.

Suddenly a spirit (through another medium) spoke out, "I am present among you." She had become possessed with the spirit "cause" of the young woman's afflictions. The spirit then spoke directly to the young woman and told her what he (the spirit) was doing to her and why. He was a spouse from a past life who was trying to convince her of his love and their unfinished relationship. He was confusing her mind and causing her distress because she had not paid attention to his attempts to communicate with her. After the president harangued the spirit to leave the young woman alone, the spirit asked the young woman to forgive him. She abandoned her rigid stance, inclined her body in the direction of the possessed medium, and said, "I forgive you." Then the first medium made *pases* over the client to take the spirit off *(despohar)*. The spirit guide-protector of the medium who was possessed by the spirit causing the woman's distress then reappeared, and the (woman) spirit gently possessed this medium in order to "refresh" and strengthen her once the *causa* spirit had departed.

At the appointed hour, or after a number of clients were served, the president initiated the final stage of the session. Prayers were again recited, including the "Our Father" and the Apostles' Creed. All of the mediums and the audience did the *despohos:* they took the distress-causing spirit beings (or their affects) off their bodies in the event that they had clung to them during the session. The ritual "opening" to receive spirit influences was thus reversed, and each human vessel was "closed" off from spirit influences with the closing of the session.

This description of a typical Spiritist healing session in Puerto Rico makes it abundantly clear that Spiritists do not consider themselves to be "healers" in the sense of taking an active role in intervening in a client's distress. They say that they "lend their bodies," which are thought of as vehicles or containers (a "material envelope") for the spirits, who do intervene. Spiritist mediums first open their bodies (including all of their senses and faculties) to receive the guide-protector spirit with whom they are currently working. This spirit presides over the work with a *causa* spirit that the medium has "seen" as responsible for a client's distress. The theme of the healer's body as a conduit is not only realized when she (or he) becomes possessed by a *guia* or *causa* spirit but also in the first stage of work with a client after the medium receives visionary evidence about the cause of her distress. She or he "captures" or "forms" (*plasmar*) that distress within her or his own body. It is very evident that the Spiritist healer's act of capturing the bodily complaints of a client she or he has never before seen (or at best has seen only a time or two), almost always without the client disclosing those complaints, brings about a feeling of immediate identification.

The only descriptive term in the literature that approximates this type of joining of feelings and bodily experiences (though not extremely well) is that of "radical empathy," which has been described as "maternal" feelings that then act as a container for a shared experience of distress (Langs, 1978). In Spiritism it takes the form of somatic identification, made possible by the healer's developed repertoire of personal, inner knowledge about illness and distress through her own suffering. This, then, is the basis for a special kind of psychological identification, a state of intimacy between healer and client that is rapidly achieved. In this state both personalities are submerged within the invisible world of spirits, where such extraordinary events are not only possible but expected. Barriers between self and other temporarily disappear (see also LeShan, 1974).

This triadic relationship (healer-client-spirit) becomes even more significant to the healing process in the event that the client is identified as being "in development" of faculties to become a healer. This occurred in an estimated 20%–25% of the over 400 sessions I observed in Puerto Rico. Persons whose distress is "seen" as caused by a guide-protector spirit trying to "come through" to the sufferer are "diagnosed" as "in development." If it is appreciated that distressful feelings (pain, somatic disturbances, confusion) place a sufferer in a one-down position of dependence on the source of relief (healer, physician, psychotherapist), then it is clear that the Spiritist healer, as the vehicle rather than the agent of change, deflects the client's dependence onto the guide-protector spirit (in this case in the guise of a distress-causing *causa* spirit). Dependence on a source of healing, in terms of lessening of distress and self-related transformation, is gradually achieved through an extended apprenticeship, working at the table during healing sessions under the protection and tutelage of one or more experienced Spiritist mediums and their protector-guide spirits. This process can take place over many healing sessions and individual consultations as the developing healer is often reluctant to take on this nomination and lifelong role.

Transcendence of inequality in the power dimension of the healing bond is an integral part of the process of "development" to become a medium-healer in Spiritism. As the novitiate healer becomes more closely linked to her or his first guide-protector, dependence on the spirit increases at the same time that dependence on a healer or other source of healing decreases and may disappear completely. Over the long term a new therapeutic bond is forged between the developing healer (formerly wounded but now "healed") and a spirit alter, who is called on to support the Spiritist medium during healing work. A special relationship forms in which the protector spirit helps the medium-healer in return for her or his attention to specific moral injunctions, obligations, and self-awareness of negative characteristics.

This more complex relationship between a "healed" client who develops as a medium-healer and spirit beings who facilitate her or his healing tasks comes full circle in the Spiritist healing ritual. Illness and distress, in the form of the *causa* spirits affecting a client, are contained by the protector spirits of the presiding mediums and thus lose their power over the client; however, the power to contain and control *does not* reside in the individual healer. Power resides in the extraordinary context of the world of the spirit. There are many implications of this type of therapeutic relationship, not the least of which is a significant shift in the locus of responsibility for the client and her or his illness (Budd & Sharma, 1994).

CONCLUSIONS: ANALOGIES BETWEEN ALTERNATIVE AND TRADITIONAL HEALING PRACTICES

If the Spiritist type of therapeutic bond (or bonds) is admitted into the model of the interpersonal aspect of the healing process, similar dimensions of other healing systems, alternative to biomedical and psychotherapeutic ones, are highlighted. In naturopathy for example, the basic notion is that of "nature cure." Power (1994) sketches the ethical implications of the perspective that the patient's healing ability, her or his natural capacity, is central to healing. The danger of a "blaming the patient" perspective is that the naturopath escapes having to take full responsibility. Power (1994) advocates a sharing of responsibility between patient and practitioner, with some sharing of power. However, when she lists images of the patient-practitioner relationship, it seems that the practitioner incorporates more powerful ones, such as "authority figure," "savior," "mother and father," and even "healer." If "nature" is thought of as an extraordinary force in the healing process, these perspectives seem contradictory and confusing for the patient.

As compared with the Spiritist model, the agency that controls change in illness in the patient appears split between patient and naturopath and nature, creating a need to clarify the role and contribution of each party to the cure. In the Spiritist case the spirits are powerful; however, healers, through responsible behavior toward personal, health- and tranquility-protecting spirits, can overcome (or redirect) illness-causing spirits. In both cases it seems that the patient/client can and perhaps must transcend dependence on a healer and learn how to assume an independent stance toward decreasing or eliminating her or his distress. In naturopathy it would seem that the role of her or his "natural capacity" for healing is the key to that process.

Davis-Floyd and Davis (1996), describing interviews with midwives, suggest that "connection" and "intuition" are central to midwifery practice and distinguish it from a biomedical, "technocratic" model. Connection is described as a web of strands connecting the mother, father, child, and midwives. It is emotional, psychic, physical, and experiential and seems to facilitate intuition in the practitioner. Intuition is defined as a special type of authoritative knowledge, a right-brained faculty distinct from "rational knowledge" (Guthrie, 1991). Midwives "learn to trust" their intuition, and it enters into their practice in unbidden ways. It is likened to an inner voice that has no sound but intrudes as needed in (usually) difficult birth situations.

Whereas intuition and spirits may seem worlds apart in any rational schematic sense, intuition could be cast as an extraordinary power in opposition to scientific explanation. In the model I have advocated as an alternative to that of the therapeutic alliance in biomedical and psychotherapeutic writings, intuition would assume the role of the third party to the therapeutic relationship between midwife and patient/family. As described by Davis-Floyd and Davis (1996), there seems to be consensual agreement among midwives about its importance as an alternative knowledge system in midwifery. However, its function as an aspect of the intimate and connected relationship between practitioner and patient in the practice of birthing is not well explicated. Its similarity to the alternative model of the therapeutic relationship outlined in this chapter is only suggestive but of definite interest in relation to how the birthing situation might be facilitated by the special connectedness that the practitioner experiences with her clients.

Naturopathy and midwifery are just two examples from a large potpourri of alternative medical systems, each with its own quasi-unique ritual or ritualized practices. The applicability of the model of therapeutic relationship I have described, derived from traditional healing practices of Latin American Spiritism as observed in Puerto Rico, must be demonstrated in a variety of medical systems. Its particular form may be highly responsive to cultural context in societies where nonvisible beings are widely accepted as ever-present, real, and viable forces in the lives of living human beings. On the other hand, an analysis of how the therapeutic relationship works in nonbiomedical healing practice is offered here in an attempt to begin to understand what the salient elements of the healing process are, regardless of modality or techniques employed across cultures.

PART V
Toward Complementary Medicine

Good ideas are not adopted automatically.
They must be driven into practice with courageous patience.
—Admiral Hyman Rickover

In Part Five we show ways in which alternative medicine is interacting with biomedicine and thereby becoming more complementary. In chapter 12, Barbara Stevens Barnum looks at how the nursing profession has been and is increasingly influenced by alternative practices. She uses nursing's most effective symbol, the "lady with the lamp," Florence Nightingale, to show how the profession is linking its origins with current practices to forge a new future. She discusses current research into the efficacy of alternative medicine and how and where alternative techniques are being taught to nurses.

As alternative practices continue to increase in popularity and biomedicine continues to try to hold its own, it is not surprising that crossover occurs, whether it is by co-optation or mutual borrowing of therapies. In chapter 13, Ronald Caplan and Wil Gesler look at a group of biomedical practitioners, MDs and DOs, who belong to the American Holistic Medical Association (AHMA). The chapter describes the origins and goals of the AHMA and provides some specific cases in which MDs are using alternative therapies. The results of a small survey of members of the AHMA are used to describe several sample characteristics.

The degree to which alternative medicine is now penetrating our educational systems is a very important measure of its current significance. In chapter 14, Evan Kligman offers medical student demands, managed care programs, and rapid changes in telecommunications as factors contributing to a substantial restructuring of curricula in many U.S. medical schools to include alternative or complementary practices. Kligman details the bases of alternative-therapy medical education programs and shows how the practice and teaching of alternative therapies are exemplified by model programs in Arizona. Added to this chapter is the personal story of an anesthesiologist who took advantage of ideas from East Asian medical philosophy and courses in alternative health care to improve his medical practice.

In chapter 15, Rena Gordon draws together the main concepts of the entire volume in six themes: (1) importance of consumer involvement, (2) changing population characteristics, (3) spatial distributions, (4) dilemmas about legitimization, (5) characteristics of the scientific community, and (6) the engine of economics. These themes can be found woven through the chapters, whose authors used different approaches in their research. Finally, Gordon uses the idea of synergy to suggest a prospective future blending of alternative medicine and biomedicine.

12

Rediscovering Nightingale: Back to the Future

Barbara Stevens Barnum

To understand what is happening today or
what will happen in the future, I look back.
—*Oliver Wendell Holmes*

This chapter looks at how the profession of nursing and alternative medicine have reciprocally interacted and affected each other. Unlike many health professions, nursing has a philosophical basis that has made acceptance of alternative therapies comfortable for many nurses. Some trace the link to the various holistic theories of nursing that gained popularity in the mid 1980s. Others say that the basis for complementary ideologies extends farther back, to the recognized founder of professional nursing, Florence Nightingale.

If we credit Nightingale with establishing roots that allow for using alternative therapies within the nursing profession, we are looking at a time frame in the mid to late 1800s. This is not to say that these roots were immediately tended. Indeed, the colorful Nightingale extended her influence in many directions, and those who followed had numerous Nightingale recommendations from which to pick and choose. Nevertheless, it seems fair to say that, for nursing, the introduction and development of complementary medicine—that is, using both alternative therapies and biomedical treatment modalities—takes us back to our origins, only to reemerge in new and interesting ways leading into our future.

Complementary medicine, thought a radical notion by many in this century, is working its way into mainstream health care as the general notion of what constitutes reality realigns. The worldview that is generally accepted in a society at any given time is termed a paradigm. A paradigm not only describes the world at any one time, it affects what is perceived and accepted as real or valid (Kuhn, 1970).

For a long time the biomedical paradigm has ruled, with its narrow boundaries concerning what phenomena could be considered "real" and what methods of discovery were acceptable. When an expanding worldview, incorporating many aspects of Eastern philosophy as well as acknowledging previously "out of bounds" phenomena, comes to be accepted, it provides a rationale for many new and revisited treatment modalities.

Nowhere are these alternative therapies more evident today than in nursing. The nursing profession, like other health professions, always reflects the trends and values of the larger society. That is why, in the era just receding, Florence Nightingale was perceived as holding the values of the scientific model of the times. Hence, Nightingale was portrayed as a sanitary engineer, an environmentalist, and a statistician—those carefully selected activities that were judged congruent with the preferred image.

In the predominant scientific era, any aspects of Nightingale's personality or preferences that were incompatible with the idealized model of reality were ignored. Nurses conveniently forgot that she eschewed the germ theory and was absorbed with aspects of spirituality that reflect many values and interests only now reemerging with today's changing paradigm. As we move into a time when the limitations of traditional science and its world ideology are being recognized, we can predict that erstwhile repressed facets of Nightingale's personality will surface—those aspects that are in keeping with the emerging paradigm. Those who wish to revamp Nightingale's image won't have to go far, for her interests were broad-ranging.

To the general public, Nightingale is generally remembered as the nurse who tackled the terrible plight of the wounded British soldiers during the Crimean War. For nurses, this is only the beginning of her many achievements. In 1853, when Sidney Herbert, the secretary for war, asked Nightingale to go to Scutari, Turkey, to care for the wounded, she was the ideal candidate for the horrendous job. Coming from a wealthy and influential family, Nightingale had (perversely, one might say) chosen a career in nursing—a job then looked on as base, ignoble, and unskilled. Having acquired what little nursing knowledge existed at the time, Nightingale was serving as superintendent of the Institute for the Care of Sick Gentlewomen in London. She left this position, assembled a cadre of nurses who met her standards, and took off for Turkey. Her efforts at establishing sanitary conditions, decreasing cholera and typhus, and cleaning up the horrible situation, resulted in a major drop in the mortality rate of the war.

Nightingale's success earned her the adoration of a nation and started her on a career of influencing health care in the British army, improving health care in India, correcting conditions in workhouses, upgrading and professionalizing nursing, and establishing the first professional school for nursing, as well as writing the first text for the teaching of nursing, *Notes on Nursing.* Her influence opened a new era in hospital reform (Schuyler, 1992).

Yet Nightingale had personal interests that ranged far beyond these pragmatic, albeit impressive, endeavors. For example, she began but did not finish writing a book on 14th-century Christian mystics. Although a lifetime Anglican, she had a long fascination with the Catholic church, possibly fueled by some of their successful nursing endeavors abroad. In truth, her notions of religion, about which she wrote frequently, do not sound much like Catholicism or Anglicanism but more like many beliefs found today. For example, her notion was of a God dwelling within the person rather than "on high" as was the typical image of her era.

Many of Nightingale's thoughts were too far-reaching for the dominant ideology of her day; they were not contained by the comfortable intellectual boxes of her times. Similarly, new theories escape beyond traditional science ideology. Although Newtonian physics still can account for middle-range physics today, it requires Einsteinian theories of relativity to explain more comprehensive phenomena. Similarly, new paradigm theories provide larger, more comprehensive explanations of reality than those accepted as "real" in the scientific paradigm. The new theories simply handle more phenomena, including various subtle aspects of health and health care. It is from this larger interpretation of reality that much of nursing's modern alternative techniques arise.

ALTERNATIVE NURSING THEORIES

Alternative nursing therapies are many and diverse at this stage, and they are not always differentiated from the therapies used by physicians and other health professionals. Ideas cutting across professional identities are among the characteristic marks of complementary medicine. Nevertheless, nurses are in the vanguard of those using the new alternative techniques. They are teaching patients to fight cancer by using visualization, lowering blood pressure through biofeedback, and using a number of other therapies such as hypnotism, therapeutic touch, aromatherapy, music therapy, acupuncture, herbal medicine, and massage, to name but a few.

Therapies that do not fit the limited scientific worldview are being adopted by many nurses, even those committed to biomedicine. Some nurses are content to accept alternative therapies simply on the basis of their efficacy. If, for example, acupuncture works, it is used even if it *should not* work according to the medical theory of cell, organ, system, and integrated body systems. If past-life therapy cures major neurotic patterns, it will be used, even if the reason it works is currently not known. At present, initial work is underway in many places to measure the effects of alternative therapies.

Many researchers have determined to investigate alternative therapies with procedures and methods approved under establishment biomedical rules. At Columbia University in New York, for example, the Complementary Care Center, founded in 1995 by a physician, Dr. Mehmet Oz, and a nurse, Mr. Jery Whitworth ("Complementary, not Alternative," 1996), tests the efficacy of alternative therapies with the rigorous tools of science. Research designs currently approved include various therapies of hypnosis, therapeutic touch, use of audiotapes, and aromatherapy, among others. All of the funded alternative therapy research projects (with a 3-year budget of just under $5 million) undergo the same rigorous scrutiny as do traditional research designs submitted to the institutional board of research review. Nurse Director Whitworth stresses the need for these alternative therapies to go mainstream as far as measurement is concerned. He and others are convinced that this is the best way for complementary medicine to reach general public and professional acceptance.

One of the first studies done by the center was a prospective, randomized, double-blind trial of the effects of hypnosis in 35 cardiac surgery patients ("Leap of Faith," 1995). Patients were randomized into two groups: those who were hypnotized and taught self-hypnosis and those who were not hypnotized. The goal was to assess whether hypnosis helped reduce the depression, pain, and discomfort associated with the surgical procedure. A standard psychological-mood inventory scale was employed, and medication use for pain and discomfort was monitored. Patients taught self-hypnosis had lower scores for the fatigue variable. Among patients receiving hypnosis education were some who did not follow through on the self-hypnosis technique postsurgery. Interestingly, this subset had the worst outcomes in terms of pain, depression, and fatigue.

Although the main goal of the center is research, it also has goals that focus on modalities that bring about the "relaxation response" and on integrating alternative and biomedical techniques into complementary medicine (see chapter 2 for the model of complementary medicine). Interestingly, one of the goals of the Complementary Care Center is to "integrate standard medical and surgical treatment with alternative medicine modalities to support and encourage the natural mechanisms that help the body recover from illness" (Complementary Care Center, 1996). This concept is not unlike that stated by Nightingale (1859/1992) in her *Notes on Nursing:* "And what nursing has to do . . . is to put the patient in the best condition for nature to act upon him" (p. 75).

Columbia is not the only major university where nurses study alternative therapies. The University of Virginia received a $1 million grant to establish the Center for the Study of Complementary and Alternative Therapies. Ann Taylor, professor of nursing and director of the center, is particularly interested in testing and using these techniques to relieve pain ("Helping People Manage Pain," 1996).

While nurses wait for the hard data to emerge on efficacy of various alternative therapies, many find it equally important to understand their underlying theories. These theories range from spiritual, metaphysical, and psychological to new physiological understandings.

Nursing's holistic perception of humans made crossing the line from the limitations of the biomedical model into the new-paradigm beliefs and prescriptions rather easy. Nursing has always claimed to care for the whole patient, not the disease. Hence, nurses were glad to accept therapies that defied the tendencies of modern science to reduce all science to a study of component parts. This is not to say that all nurses crossed the line into holistic methods.

As segments of nursing moved in the direction of using alternative therapies, several disparate interpretations of new-paradigm nursing emerged. In one view, typified by Newman (1994), mind (not brain), in the form of expanded consciousness, is what truly comprises humans; and nursing's mission is to assist people to expand their consciousness. In another view, typified by Dossey and her colleagues (Dossey, Keegan, Guzzetta, & Kolkmeier, 1995), spirit was added as a new component of humans, an element that was different from, not a substitute for, the previously defined biopsychosocial elements. In this image, nursing simply added one more task to its roster: care of the spirit. In other theories, typified by Watson (1988), a spiritual interpretation prevailed in which a human being was a soul vulnerable to disharmony, a state that could result in illness. Here the nurse's task was one of restoring the soul's harmony so that the illness could be cured.

None of these notions cast the nurse in the physiologically based role that is still typical of how nursing is seen today by most nurses. However, there is a strong attempt to justify holistic therapeutics according to newer physiological knowledge and hypotheses. Dossey et al. (1995), for example, offer this explanation for the body-mind linkage:

> New ideas and events evoke bodymind changes; that is, neural pathways and consciousness connect to permit information transduction. For example, a hypertensive client may believe that cold hands are a normal part of her physiology. As she begins to monitor hand temperature on awakening and throughout the day, however, a pattern begins to emerge. Her hands are usually warm on awakening, but become cold in response to daily stressors/ activities. As she learns handwarming techniques, breathing exercises, and other bodymind interventions, the client has a first-hand experience of information transduction. (p. 89)

In part, Dossey et al. (1995) relate holistic therapies to autonomic responses, citing stages in which images, thoughts, attitudes, and feelings from the
frontal cortex are transmitted by the neurotransmitters norepinephrine and
acetylcholine to organ systems and autonomic nervous system branches.
With this conception, the mind modulates the biochemical function throughout the autonomic nervous system, producing a connection between images,
feelings, emotions, spirit, and their physiology or pathophysiology. In similar fashion, Dossey et al. describe links between mind and the endocrine
system (the mind-gene connection, as Dossey calls it), the immune system,
and the neuropeptide system (pp. 97–107).

This approach, currently coming into fashion in nursing and other fields,
allows for the claim that holistic medicine is truly complementary to biomedicine, its effectiveness traceable to new scientific data just emerging
about mind, spirit, and body interconnections. Nor is the interconnection a
one-way street; body can affect mind or spirit just as the mind can have
effects in the opposite direction.

Thus, these newer, alternative views of reality involve major reconcep-
tualizations of nursing therapeutics as well as different perceptions of what
it means to be a human being. However they are described, the underlying
paradigms share some or all of the following assumptions:

1. A person's thoughts have greater impact on her or his body than was
conceptualized in the older psychosomatic models. Techniques such as
visualization (guided imagery) may be used for healing because they can
reprogram the body as well as the mind.

2. The body holds or stores emotions and events in various body parts,
and these emotions may be affected through forms of body work, such as
massage. Massage may be delivered by techniques such as deep muscle
manipulation in rolfing or by reflexology, a system that uses acupressure
points and massage of the feet, which are seen as having discrete parts corresponding with and affecting specific body organs and parts. Sometimes
massage is combined with various forms of psychotherapy.

3. The human being extends beyond her or his visible tactile body to
include different layers of an etheric body (aura) that begins where one's
skin leaves off. These energy layers have different vibratory frequencies
and properties, and together they create an aura that influences health. Auric
levels may give evidence of disease before body changes become apparent. The aura may be manipulated by the knowledgeable nurse to prevent
incipient illness.

4. Personal energy and/or a universal energy exist(s) and may be tapped
for healing. Therapeutic touch and other manipulations of energy (such as
reiki) may be used to deliver this energy to patients requiring it.

NURSING APPLICATIONS: WHERE AND HOW

Alternative nursing therapies are taught to nurses in two educational designs. Some education programs add alternative therapies (usually at the master's level) to program content primarily presented in the standard curricula. Other master's degree programs, usually labeled as holistic nursing programs, focus exclusively on therapies falling within the new paradigm. Holistic complementary therapy programs or units of study can be found across the United States, from the University of Colorado, Denver, in the West, to the College of New Rochelle, New Rochelle, New York, in the East.

Gold and Anastasi (1995) identified numerous programs open to nurses interested in studying holistic modalities, including schools of nursing at Adelphi University, the College of New Rochelle, Florida Atlantic University, and the University of Louisville. In addition, they identify various education programs offered specifically for nurses by the American Holistic Nursing Association, Esalen Institute, Holistic Nursing Associates, the New Center for Wholistic Health Education and Research, the New York Open Center, and the Omega Institute, as well as new paradigm therapy programs shared with other practitioners.

In nursing practice settings, distribution of alternative therapies shows as wide a dispersion as occurs in nursing education settings. Additionally, alternative therapies are used in traditional settings, along with routine medicine and nursing care (such as the relaxation sessions and regular healing circles for nurses used at Beth Israel Medical Center in New York City), and in nursing centers that specialize in alternative therapies (such as Holistic Nursing Consultants of Santa Fe, New Mexico, or the Wholistic Health Center in Syosset, New York). Combinations of biomedicine and alternative medicine are growing more commonplace as practitioners in various professions give up their resistance to alternative therapies.

At present there is no organized way to estimate the increase in use of alternative therapies among nurses. However, alternative therapies clearly have found their way into nursing's traditional scholarly paths. Professional nursing has several journals dedicated to alternative therapies (e.g., *Alternative Health Practitioner* and *Holistic Nursing Practice*) as well as complementary care articles that appear with increasing frequency in the more traditional nursing journals. Take, for example, the recent article comparing nurses and alternative healers (Engebretson, 1996) in the research journal *Image* or an article on shifting mainstream medicine in the more widely distributed newspaper, *Nursing Spectrum* (Steefel, 1996).

There are at present few data to gauge the extent of alternative practices. The National League for Nursing, for example, does not differentiate approved schools according to whether or not their curricula are holistic.

The general impression of the author is that one does not need to sample many schools or care institutions before finding evidence of complementary practices. The American Holistic Nurses Association gives "official" status to the new approach. The organization's growth has been remarkable. It now reports a membership of approximately 4,650 nurses. More interesting, its membership has been growing in the past few years by 75 to 100 members per month.

RATIONALE FOR METHODS

In nursing, therapies are sometimes differentiated on the basis of doing and being (Dossey et al., 1995), namely:

> Doing therapies include almost all forms of modern medicine, such as medications, procedures, dietary manipulations, radiation, and acupuncture. In contrast, being therapies do not employ things but utilize states of consciousness, such as imagery, prayer, meditation, and quiet contemplation, as well as the presence and intention of the nurse. These techniques are therapeutic because of the power of the psyche to affect the body. (p. 14)

Although some alternative therapies, such as acupuncture, may fall within the "doing" side, many (such as guided imagery) fall in the newer "being" category. Others, like energy movement, may combine both elements.

Dossey and her colleagues (1995) further differentiate the sources of these methods as falling on two ends of a healing spectrum, rational and paradoxical:

> "Doing" therapies fall into the rational healing category, because they make sense to our linear, intellectual thought processes. . . . On the other hand, `being' therapies fall into the paradoxical healing category, because they frequently happen without a scientific explanation. A paradox is a seemingly absurd or contradictory statement or event that is, in fact, true." (pp. 16–17)

This division of the nurse's role into doing and being conveniently adds a new component to older therapies without negating them. In addition to cure work, the new therapies may involve creating a state of transcendence in which the outcome of the disease process is less important and, indeed, is surmounted by a spiritual recovery/enhancement.

One finds the entire gamut of alternative therapies used by nurses, including energy movement, massage, reflexology, hypnosis, guided imagery, biofeedback, acupuncture, herbal therapy, aromatherapy, and music therapy, among others. Yet the profession seems to have developed its own favorites, among them energy work (particularly therapeutic touch) and guided imagery. These will be looked at briefly.

ENERGY WORK

In nursing, many of the new paradigm therapies involve methods of moving energy and altering the patient's energy field. Two possible notions of energy are seen at work here; in some systems, only the human energy fields (of nurse and patient) are considered and manipulated. In other systems, a universal energy is proposed to exist and to be accessible to manipulations.

As indicated earlier, the human energy field is conceived as extending beyond the physical body in vibratory layers of energy (termed the human aura), visible to some, but not all, persons. These layers of being are neither accepted nor researched in the scientific model. Those who claim the existence of these energy layers see them as mediating numerous aspects of the person's existence, including health and illness manifestations.

Reiki, core energetics, and other common energy manipulation systems are used by nurses to influence health. The most common application is therapeutic touch, in which the nurse conveys energy from her hands to the patient. Therapeutic touch was introduced into nursing by Krieger (1979), who observed the use of the technique in other cultures. Therapeutic touch is widely taught now throughout North America. Krieger's original concept was based on the transmission of the nurse's own excess energy. Krieger (1981) says about *prana* (energy):

> I saw the healer to be an individual whose personal health gave him or her access to an overabundance of prana (the healer's health being an indication that he or she was in highly efficient interaction with the significant field forces) and whose motivation and intentionality gave him or her a certain control over the projection of prana for the well-being of others. (p. 143)

Keegan (in Dossey et al., 1995) describes the phases of therapeutic touch as follows:

1. centering oneself physically and psychologically; that is, finding within oneself an inner reference of stability;
2. exercising the natural sensitivity of the hand to assess the energy field of the client for clues to differentiate the quality of energy flow;
3. mobilizing areas in the client's energy field that appear to be non-flowing (i.e., sluggish, congested, or static);
4. directing one's own excess body energies to assist the client to repattern his or her own energies. (p. 548)

In contrast to these explanations, other proponents of moving energy (such as *reiki* practitioners) claim to draw on universal energy rather than on their own. Typically, they describe four major steps: (1) centering within oneself so that one is detached from outside interference, thoughts, or negativities; (2) grounding oneself in an energy source outside of oneself in such a way that one can tap that universal energy; (3) focusing that energy through oneself to the patient, so as not to draw on one's own bodily energy; and (4) intention, that is, employing the will and affect so as to intend a good effect for the patient. Nurses sometimes refer to these tactics as repatterning.

Quinn (1994) describes the altered states required:

> At the start of a Therapeutic Touch session the nurse centers, that is, turns his or her attention inward, reaching a calm, relaxed, and open state of consciousness. In this state of consciousness, the Therapeutic Touch practitioner then consciously formulates the intent to be an instrument for helping or healing and focuses on wholeness and balance in the recipient. This process on the part of the Therapeutic Touch practitioner may be thought of as a repatterning of his or her own energy field in the direction of expanded consciousness, a consciousness experienced as unified, harmonious, peaceful, and ordered. (p. 66)

Some practitioners theorize that altered states of consciousness underlie these practices of centering, grounding, focusing, and intentionality. It may be that energy work draws on abilities for which we may one day have a descriptive science, a science that measures levels and states of consciousness as well as levels and kinds of energy transmitted. Such a science would eventually correlate levels and states of consciousness with their particular energy effects.

Energy work, however described, tends to address new techniques, altered states of consciousness, and altered sensitivities to subtle phenomena not usually perceived. Brennan (1988) calls the latter *high sense perception,* and it involves visual, sensate, and other perceptive modalities that give information concerning the status of a person's energy field. The different systems of energy work may deal with one, two, or all three of these elements (techniques, altered states, and perceptions).

Whatever the differences in approach and philosophy, energy work is one of nursing's favorite tools. The use of guided imagery is also very popular, probably second only to therapeutic touch in common use within the profession.

Guided Imagery

Krieger (1981), Dossey et al. (1995), and many other nurses use guided imagery in at least two separate ways. In the first use a nurse might have a patient mentally practice how he or she will perform health-related activities. For example, a patient might rehearse how he or she will manage morning activities of daily living (ADL) when going home after a stroke that caused loss of some functions. In essence, visualization is used here as mental practice. It may involve motivation, psychological adjustment, or actual aspects of learning.

The second use of guided imagery is the attempt to "program" a patient (including her or his body) to fight a disease, such as is done in cancer therapy. Many people have a simplistic notion of guided imagery: for example, a patient imagines (visualizes) his or her body's cells attacking and destroying cancer cells. This is not to say that such simple use of imagery is not of value, but the technique has a more complex basis and more facets than this simple example illustrates. Dossey et al. (1995) describe it this way: "Imagery is not about mental pictures, but is a resource for gaining access to the imagination and more subtle aspects of inner experience. It may involve all sensory modalities: visual, olfactory, tactile, gustatory, auditory, and kinesthetic" (p. 611).

OTHER THERAPIES

Although therapeutic touch and guided imagery are possibly the most common nursing practices, individual nurse practitioners draw on techniques in all three alternative sections of the model presented in chapter 2. From the cross-cultural quadrant, they use yoga and Chinese acupuncture; from the mind/spirit quadrant, they use hypnotherapy, visualization, and meditation; and from the body healing quadrant, they use massage, aromatherapy, nutrition counseling, and herbal therapies, to name but a few.

Interestingly, adaptation and application of methods residing outside biomedicine are not the privilege of any particular profession. The same alternative treatments are being applied by many and varied professionals. This "leveling" of erstwhile separate professions through the use of the same techniques seems appropriate to complementary therapy, making for more holistic health practitioners as well as for more holistic health practices.

Two trends in nursing are operating at the same time. Although alternative therapies are not exclusive to nursing, they reinforce a change that was already taking place in traditional scientific nursing, that is, a movement from a caring model to a curing ideology. At one stage, nursing and medicine were conveniently differentiated by the claim that medicine cured the disease while nursing cared for the person with the disease. That differentiation died within the biomedical model as nurse practitioners entered primary care and took on "curing" tasks.

Many alternative treatments also aim at curing rather than caring. Therapeutic touch, for example, is conceived as potentially relieving various illness states. Similarly, biofeedback might be used to cure high blood pressure. Often the newer term, *healing*, has been substituted for the older one, *curing*.

This allows for a subtle shift in image to healing the person rather than curing the disease. As we saw in many of the nursing models employing alternative therapies, healing the person may have more to do with psychological and spiritual states than with the disease.

NEW PARADIGM AND SCIENCE: A RECONCILIATION?

It is interesting to observe that each major age (and its worldview) is replaced by a differing perception of reality. Despite negating the worldview that recedes before it, each era incorporates much of that era into it. Hence, in the present trend, one finds alternative practitioners attempting to justify their effects by the best of scientific research or seeking to explain the physiological basis for the effectiveness of their practices through rigorous scientific demonstration. New-paradigm practitioners generally accept the work of science, including modern medical applications. An ideological shift toward cooperation rather than competition between the two schools of thought also is taking place.

As new domains of inquiry and new therapies become acceptable, nursing, like other professions, will rewrite its history to incorporate these changes. No doubt, part of the change will be retrospective, reaching back into nursing's history. It is predictable that those heretofore unacceptable aspects of personality and behavior of the discipline's leader and founder, Nightingale, will be acknowledged instead of selectively ignored. Once again, we will recognize the emotive, one might even say holistic, image of the "lady with the lamp." The historical image of Nightingale—walking the aisles between cots of wounded soldiers in Crimea, holding her lamp high, raising the hopes and recovery rate of the wounded soldiers—will once again be acceptable to the profession. No doubt, someone will describe her effect as "being" rather than "doing" therapy, realigning Nightingale's image to fit the predominant notion of reality.

13

Biomedical Physicians Practicing Holistic Medicine

Ronald L. Caplan and Wilbert M. Gesler

Doctors think a lot of patients are cured who have simply quit in disgust.
—*Don Herold*

Americans exercise their right to choose among competing forms of health care (Gevitz, 1988), utilizing practitioners from medical systems with differing beliefs about illness and health. Throughout this book the choice among practitioners is illustrated by a four-part model of complementary medicine that categorizes specific practices as either biomedicine or one of three types of alternative medicine. Boundaries between parts are blurring, however, as an increasing number of biomedical physicians use alternative therapies and holistic concepts in their medical practice.

Holistic medicine is best defined as "an informal collection of attitudes and practices, not a defined system of treatment" (Weil, 1995, p. 180). Several main concepts of holistic medicine include body balance; energy; physical, mental, and emotional wellness; self-healing; equality of the healer-patient relationship; social and cultural context; and low-tech remedies. Practitioners of alternative medicine generally use holistic concepts in their healing. For example, several of the better known alternative therapies, such as homeopathy and naturopathy, can be considered holistic. Holistic tenets also are held by practitioners within such major cross-cultural and ethnic medical systems as Chinese and Ayurvedic. It is clear that these concepts cut across boundaries of alternative medicine sectors in the complementary medicine model. The focus of this chapter is the group of physicians trained in biomedicine who practice holistic medicine.

Over the past two decades, Americans have steadily increased their use of alternative practitioners, including many holistic medical doctors (Caplan & Scarpaci, 1989). As the public's demand for alternative health care has increased, professional interest has grown in both alternative practices and holistic concepts of health. For example, in 1977 several thousand doctors attended an Association for Holistic Health conference in San Diego. The following year the American Holistic Medical Association (AHMA) was founded by "a group of physicians who felt the need for an organized forum to explore and promote holistic health care" (AHMA, 1996). In 1996, 600 self-described holistic MDs and DOs and their students were members of that association. Other health care practitioners may join as associate members. This number does not represent all holistic physicians and students in the country. Although the total number is unknown, it is suspected that it is greater than the reported 600.

According to its mission statement, the AHMA (1996) aims "to support practitioners in their evolving personal and professional development and to promote an art and science which acknowledges all aspects of the individual, the family and the planet." In defining holistic health, the AHMA emphasizes the following: health as more than the mere absence of disease; environmental, mental, emotional, social, and spiritual as well as physical health; a partnership between patient and physician; and the importance of both prevention and cure. More specifically, the AHMA stresses the following: educating people about lifestyle changes and self-care; using complementary approaches as well as conventional surgery and drugs; finding out what kind of patient has a disease as well as what disease a patient has; recognizing that illness represents a dysfunction of the whole person rather than an isolated event; viewing illness, pain, and dying as learning opportunities; and encouraging patients to use love, hope, and humor and to drive out hate, despair, and grief.

The American Board of Holistic Medicine was set up by AHMA members to certify physicians as practitioners of holistic medicine. The board examination covers seven core areas: nutrition, physical activity, environmental medicine, behavioral medicine, social health, energy medicine, and spiritual attunement. In addition, the examination covers six secondary areas: botanical medicine, homeopathy, ethnomedicine (traditional Chinese medicine, Ayurveda, Native American medicine), manual medicine (manipulation, body work), biomolecular therapies, and health promotion. The association also hosts an annual conference; publishes a quarterly journal, *Holistic Medicine,* as well as monographs on holistic medicine; has committees working on specific issues; and provides student support.

The federal government also is investigating holistic health care. As early as 1979 the Department of Health, Education and Welfare sponsored a conference—"Holistic Health: A Public Policy." More recently, the National Institutes of Health established an Office of Alternative Medicine (OAM), also discussed in chapters 1, 3, and 14. Clearly, the alternative health care movement "is not limited to a handful of zealots in California, as is often assumed, but is truly nationwide" (Rosch, 1981, p. 60).

The growth of holistic health care represents an important and relatively recent trend in American medicine, away from the reductionist concepts of biomedicine and toward more holistic concepts. This shift is usually thought of in terms of a dichotomy: a health care practitioner is or is not part of the biomedical system. Many people may think that holistic practitioners are constantly competing with and trying to replace their biomedical counterparts, while at the same time biomedical practitioners are trying to eliminate them. This kind of competition between the two types of health care is no doubt occurring and perhaps even intensifying. However, the shift in American health care toward more holistic or "natural" remedies is also taking place within biomedicine itself. There appears to be a growing number of biomedical practitioners who are also holistic. Consequently, the boundary between the two systems is breaking down, and there is now a significant amount of overlap between them.

One way to demonstrate that the edges of the model are blurring is to look at what people trained in biomedicine think about practitioners of other forms of health care. Some think that most, if not all of them, are quacks and should be outlawed (Glymour & Stalker, 1983). At the other extreme are those practitioners who have largely abandoned the theories and practices of biomedicine (Gordon, 1980). An increasing number of medical doctors appear to be somewhere in the middle (McKeown, 1993). After interviewing 250 medical doctors, the authors of a recently published book conclude that the medical profession is not nearly as opposed to alternative therapies as it was 10 years ago (Janiger & Goldberg, 1994).

A recent British study provides a more detailed analysis of medical opinions about alternative health care. Perkin and his colleagues (Perkin, Pearcy, & Fraser, 1994) sent a questionnaire to a random sample of 100 general practitioners (GPs) and 100 hospital doctors in the South West Thames Regional Health Authority and to a convenience sample of 237 preclinical medical students at St. George's Hospital Medical School. The questionnaire asked respondents to rate their attitude toward alternative medicine from 1 (no interest) to 10 (active interest) and to answer several other questions about alternative health care. The results showed that alternative medicine was quite popular among medical students (mean rating, 6.0) and GPs (mean rating, 5.5); not as much interest was shown by hospital doctors (mean rating, 4.3). The study in this part of England showed that feelings were fairly positive toward alternative health care, although not all types of practitioners were equally enthusiastic. This study also reported that a substantial proportion of its respondents (12% of hospital doctors and 20% of GPs) were practicing alternative therapies.

The authors of this chapter decided that one way to explore the holistic/biomedical overlap in the United States was to study a group of medical doctors (MDs) who practice holistic health care. Because members of the AHMA were, by definition representative of the overlap, attention was focused on them.

Why is it important to study these holistic MDs and DOs? For a start, we would like to know what kind of people they are, especially in comparison to their nonholistic practicing colleagues. How do they differ from nonholistic MDs and DOs in terms of gender, age, and income? What are some of the basic characteristics of their practices? How do they get along with other health care practitioners? Concerning their medical futures, what are their greatest hopes and fears? The answers to these types of questions can help us better understand the future consequences of the current trend in American health care. More specifically, we would also gain some important insights into emerging crossover forms of health care that combine the best of both systems or, alternatively, that reveal irreconcilable differences. Will conflict or integration characterize American health care at the beginning of the next century?

The following section of this chapter examines some recent investigations of biomedical physicians who use holistic therapies in their practice, including our own survey of AHMA members. The chapter concludes with a brief discussion of the future of holistic health care in the United States.

PHYSICIANS WHO PRACTICE HOLISTIC MEDICINE

As noted earlier, the total number of holistic biomedical physicians (MDs and DOs) in the United States is unknown. One problem is the absence of a widely agreed on definition of holistic medicine. A study of physicians who practice holistic medicine (Goldstein, Sutherland, Jaffe, & Wilson, 1987, 1988) surveyed 340 members of the AHMA and 142 family practitioners (FPs) who were not members and compared their demographic, educational, and practice characteristics. Both groups were asked to rate the value of 25 holistic practices, such as meditation/realization, acupuncture, massage/rolfing, and iridology. Although there was considerable variation within each group, the holistic group's ratings were statistically significantly higher for 22 of the 25 practices. However, the techniques used most frequently by the AHMA members were also quite widely used by the nonholistic FPs. It was also found that "items which reflect more emotional involvement, a more equal relationship, and less reliance on traditional barriers between physicians and their clients exhibit the greatest differences" (Goldstein et al., 1988, p. 858).

Of interest in these findings is that the two groups differed a great deal in their personal lives. For example, AHMA members were twice as likely as FPs to state that religious or spiritual experiences influenced their lives and views on health. They were also much more likely to promote their own health by using such techniques as exercise or meditation. Despite these results, Goldstein and his colleagues (1987, 1988) concluded that there were surprisingly few differences between holistic MDs and mainstream medicine (at least the type practiced by FPs). The substantial overlap between these two samples of biomedical physicians supports the claim that a shift in American medicine is indeed occurring. Furthermore, they predicted more integration in the future, at least in some areas of medical practice.

There is some evidence that these predictions are coming true. As more of its practitioners employ holistic therapies, biomedicine increasingly becomes more holistic. For example, Dr. Memet Oz, a cardiothoracic surgeon at Columbia-Presbyterian Medical Center in New York City, is a pioneer in this area (Brown, 1995). As an expertly trained surgeon, he was dissatisfied with elements of his practice. He could not change the pathogenic lifestyles of his patients, which all too often put them on the operating table in the first place. He also wanted to enlist patients' emotional and psychological energy in the healing process. In an effort to accomplish both objectives, he established the Complementary Care Center. This center advocates the use of diet, meditation and hypnosis, therapeutic massage, and the energy medicine of hands-on healers to promote healing. Dr. Oz has found that patients who were taught self-hypnosis were less tense, less depressed, and less tired after surgery than those who had not received this training (see also chapters 12 and 14).

Dr. Oz is not alone. Frustrated by the many limitations and unanswered questions of biomedicine, many of its practitioners have embraced alternative therapies, if not for their patients then for themselves and their families (Janiger & Goldberg, 1994; Moskowitz, 1993). Perhaps the best known is Dr. Andrew Weil (1995), who in his best-selling book, *Spontaneous Healing*, explains that his search for alternatives started over 20 years ago in the Amazon rain forest. Many of the allied health professionals, such as physical therapists, are also more accepting of alternative therapies (McLaughlin, 1995).

In May 1996 the World Congress on Complementary Therapies in Medicine held a 3-day conference in Washington, DC, chaired by Dr. C. Everett

Koop, Senior Scholar at the Everett Koop Institute at Dartmouth and former Surgeon General. Participants examined several alternative health care approaches that could become part of integrated healthcare systems. The keynote speaker was Dr. Dean Ornish, who spoke about the use of diet, exercise, and meditation to reverse coronary heart disease. Other topics discussed were nutritional medicine, Chinese medicine, naturopathy, and complementary medicine in cancer care and AIDS.

EXPLORATORY CASE STUDY OF HOLISTIC MDS

In 1989, Ron Caplan and Wil Gesler surveyed the entire 1988 membership list of AHMA, which totals around 200 holistic biomedical physicians. Their target population was all physicians (both MDs and DOs) listed in the 1988 directory of the AHMA who were in active, direct patient practice in the United States (they excluded members outside the United States). Eighty-nine usable questionnaires were returned, resulting in a response rate of 44.9%. Reported here are only those items most closely related to the overlap between biomedicine and holistic health care.

GEOGRAPHIC DISTRIBUTION

The proportion of all physicians belonging to the AHMA (209 in total) in each of the four U.S. census regions was compared with the expected proportion based on the distribution of all nonfederal physicians. The West clearly had substantially more members than expected. The Northeast was somewhat underrepresented, the North Central region achieved near parity, and the South was the most underrepresented.

These results indicate that, in respect to having holistic physicians, the West was relatively innovative, whereas the South was relatively conservative. Furthermore, the widespread perception that holistic health care is primarily confined to some eccentrics in California was not supported.

PERSONAL CHARACTERISTICS

Do AHMA members possess personal traits that somehow set them apart or that could be used to establish a profile of a holistic MD? Compared to all physicians in the United States, there were fewer AHMA members in the youngest (<35 years) and the oldest (65+) age groups but more in between (35–64). Perhaps older MDs have had little exposure to holism or are more reluctant to try new therapies. In contrast, younger physicians may still be strongly influenced by their medical training and hesitant to deviate from it. They also lack sufficient practical experience. On the other hand, middle-aged physicians may have just enough frustration and confidence to try something new.

With respect to gender, the sample of holistic practitioners did not differ from the general population of MDs. Given the prevailing notion that women are more caring than men, one might think that women would be more likely to employ alternative therapies than men would. However, this gender-biased stereotype was not supported by our study (admittedly based on small numbers).

According to the study results, holistic MDs earn approximately the same income as their nonholistic counterparts when medical specialties are taken into account. For example, their median income, after expenses but before taxes, was $76,970. Median net income for all United States physicians in general and family practice in 1987 was $80,000; and for pediatricians it was $77,000 (Gonzalez & Emmons, 1988). In 1987 median net income for United States physicians in *all* specialties was $108,000. Study respondents appear to be on the lower end of the earnings scale, receiving salaries on a par with pediatricians, GPs, and FPs.

HOLISTIC ASPECTS OF PRACTICE

In the study population the mean number of years practicing holistic medicine was 10.8, and the median number of years was 9. When asked to what extent their current practice was holistic, about two thirds identified strongly with the holistic label, and the other third acknowledged the label to some degree. When asked, "How much more satisfied with your practice are you since becoming a 'holistic' practitioner?" 69.2% (54) replied "very much," and 30.8% (24) said "somewhat," a relatively high level of satisfaction and optimism.

RELATIONS WITH OTHER HEALTH CARE PRACTITIONERS

Because the survey targeted a group of practitioners at the interface between alternative medicine and biomedicine, they were asked about their relationships with three other types of practitioners: nonholistic MDs, other holistic MDs, and alternative healers such as chiropractors, naturopaths, and homeopaths. Relationships were clearly the best with other holistic MDs and worst with nonholistic MDs, with alternative healers somewhere in the middle. Perhaps regular MDs disapprove of these holistic hybrids and seek to distance themselves from them, the proverbial "other." On the other hand, alternative practitioners appear to be more welcoming. This finding could illustrate the system shift discussed above, with innovators within the biomedical profession moving away from their origins and toward a more hospitable alternative.

Based on the study results, holistic MDs are fairly bullish about their future (see Figure 13.1). About two thirds of them (39.0% + 27.3%) thought that their practices had a good to excellent chance of expanding over the next 5 years. The remaining third had some doubts. Approximately half of the respondents (21.1% + 28.9%) thought that holistic medicine would be more integrated with biomedicine in the future. The other half rated the chances of such an integration as fair to poor, reflecting their skepticism about biomedicine changing enough to include them. Most saw a continuing split between alternative and biomedical practitioners. Only one fourth of the respondents (26.0%) thought that holistic doctors would be more integrated with other alternative practitioners over the next 5 years. A third rated the chances of such integration as fair. And a full two fifths thought it was unlikely.

Following a shift in medical care, one would expect a period of compromise and integration. Because the respondents did not see this happening any time soon, this shift in American health care is probably far from over.

CONCLUSION

Despite the efforts of the AMA and the pharmaceutical industry to stop it (Caplan, 1988; Lisa, 1994), the integration of holistic and mainstream medicines not only will continue but most likely will accelerate. As frustrated physicians become more receptive and holistic practitioners become more popular, the boundaries between them will increasingly blur and their overlaps will expand.

During the 1980s the principal integrating force was the *pull* (i.e., attraction) of holistic therapies on a relatively small but growing number of biomedical practitioners. They were dissatisfied with their practices and were actively seeking holistic therapies. For the most part, they were the overlap between biomedicine and holistic health care, and a sample of this group comprised the study population for the case study described.

In the early 1990s another force came, from outside medicine, and brought biomedicine and holistic health care closer together. This force, more powerful than the pull of holistic therapies on frustrated physicians, was the *push* of government, insurance companies, and health maintenance organizations (HMOs). In an effort to lower costs and improve quality, some large payers of medical care have begun paying for selected

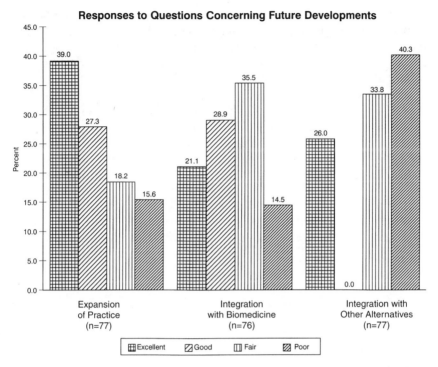

FIGURE 13.1 Responses to questions on future developments in holistic practice.

alternative therapies, which include holistic concepts such as naturopathy, reflexology, and homeopathy (Cowley et al., 1995). They consider these alternatives to biomedicine to be safer, cheaper, and in many cases, customer-preferred (Mitchell, 1993).

Three examples, one for each payer, are given. With respect to government, Seattle will soon establish a naturopathic health clinic (Egan, 1996; see also chapter 6, this volume). It will be supported by tax revenues and employ both naturopaths and medical physicians. It also will be the country's first such clinic. In the insurance industry, companies like Prudential, the Seattle-based Health Cooperative of Puget Sound, and Mutual of Omaha now cover, respectively, acupuncture, midwife-assisted home births, and low-fat vegetarian diets for heart disease patients (Baar, 1995; Peltz, 1993). Finally, many HMOs, including one of the nation's fastest growing (Oxford Health Plans), are allowing enrollees to choose alternative healers, such as naturopaths and homeopaths, as their primary care physicians (Baar, 1995).

These two forces—the pull of holistic therapies and the push by government, insurance companies, and HMOs—will be a powerful combination.

Over time, all this pushing and pulling will undoubtedly bring holistic health care and biomedicine closer together. They may even gradually replace decades of competition and hostility with a new era of cooperation and trust. Such a transformation of American health care would greatly benefit all its practitioners and their patients.

14

Medical Education: Changes and Responses

Evan W. Kligman

Education's purpose is to replace an empty mind with an open one.
—Malcolm S. Forbes

A lternative medicine has emerged as an important new curricular component of mainstream medical education. Over 30 medical schools, among the most prestigious in the United States, have developed substantive courses in alternative (complementary, integrative) medicine. Medical education is responding to the same external and internal forces, mentioned in earlier chapters, that are making an impact on the delivery of health care in this country. To reiterate, these forces include changing demographics (e.g., the maturing of baby boomers); a growing orientation toward health promotion and natural treatments; managed care and marketplace health care reform; telecommunications and the Internet; growing interest among the public, medical students, and practicing physicians; growth in the work force of alternative medicine clinicians; and private and federal support for state-of-the-art research in alternative therapies.

ALTERNATIVE MEDICINE: REEMERGENCE IN MEDICAL EDUCATION

Modern biomedical education evolved as a reaction to an eclectic environment of approaches and varying medical philosophies of health and disease prominent over 100 years ago. As we embark on the 21st century, there are over 150 recognized alternative therapies typically considered out of the realm of Western medicine traditions and not part of the core curriculum taught in most American allopathic or osteopathic medical schools.

Many of these therapies were commonplace a century ago, prior to the Flexner Report of 1910 and the standardization of medical education. Indeed, some of these therapies, such as homeopathy and chiropractic, were considered not only safer but more efficacious than the allopathic care delivered before medical education became based on the biomedical paradigm.

Over the past 15 years there has been a remarkable surge in interest, among both the public and the medical communities, in alternative and complementary forms of health care (Monson, 1995). Some studies have shown that 80% of medical residents in the United States and Canada want some training in alternative medicine, and a survey of primary care physicians revealed that 80% were interested in learning more about at least one alternative therapy. In a 1994 study of how allopathic physicians participate in the decision to refer patients for alternative therapies, more than 60% of all physicians were found to have made referrals to alternative providers at least once in the preceding year, 38% in the preceding month (Borkan et al., 1994). An article in the *Journal of the Royal Society of Medicine* revealed that 93% of British general practitioners had, on at least one occasion, suggested a referral for alternative treatment (Hansen, 1991). Another study surveyed around 300 family physicians in New England, with more than 90% considering alternative medical therapies as legitimate medical practices. Further, most of the physicians desired training in various alternative therapies (Berman et al., 1995).

Indeed, new programs are developing each year in the most prestigious United States medical schools, some of which are evolving toward a synthesis called integrative medicine (Weil, 1995). It is commonplace also to see several books on the best-seller list covering one form or another of alternative therapies. Jerry M. Calkins, MD, PhD, has provided the following case study.

ACUPUNCTURE IN PAIN MANAGEMENT: A PHYSICIAN'S PERSPECTIVE

As a practicing anesthesiologist with interests in surgical and acute and chronic pain management, I have treated patients suffering from acute and chronic pain who have not responded to anything that I, as an allopathic physician, could recommend or offer. My inability to help patients at times left me frustrated and in search of alternatives. In this search for methods of treating these most complex and difficult cases, I became aware of other traditional systems of health care.

In pursuit of education and training in alternative concepts, I have begun to appreciate the integral relationship of humankind with the universe. The biological, chemical, and physical laws of nature that govern our existence are maintained throughout the universe in an integrated, harmonious fashion. When we live in harmony with our world, we are well. It is the disharmony of our patients with their environment that challenges us as physicians to recall that the practice of medicine is more than a science. It is also the art of healing that enables the patient to reestablish the harmony of her or his life.

A colleague of mine introduced me to the philosophical approaches to medicine of the Far East and to traditional Chinese medicine (TCM) in particular. As I began to develop an understanding of and appreciation for TCM and for medical acupuncture in particular, I became acutely aware of the fact that we as Western physicians are naive to think that Western allopathic and osteopathic medicine provide the panacea of health care. Many of us in Western biomedicine were taught a very mechanistic approach to life and health. For example, we learned that a heart is a pump and the lungs are gas exchangers. As an allopathic physician, I am able to offer the patient a pill, surgery, or a psychiatrist. My osteopathic colleagues add a fourth modality, osteopathic manipulation.

However, there are many types of health care delivery systems in the world, each with its successes and failures. From my own experience, those patients who are failed by one system sometimes find successful therapy in another. Such is the case in the utilization of medical acupuncture in an allopathic practice.

To become an effective practitioner of the healing arts, I have had to become knowledgeable in other systems of health care and have had to learn how to integrate them into my medical practice. I received my training in medical acupuncture through the Medical Acupuncture for Physicians course under the direction of Joseph Helms, MD, and sponsored by the UCLA School of Medicine and the American Academy of Medical Acupuncture (AAMA). The AAMA was established to promote education and principles of practice for physician acupuncturists. This organization has been instrumental in developing basic and advanced educational programs for physicians, public education, and referral services, as well as addressing physician concerns regarding hospital privileges, malpractice insurance coverage, and third-party insurance reimbursement. In addition to the AAMA, the American Foundation of Medical Acupuncture (AFMA) has been established to promote research in scientific and clinical arenas.

I am not suggesting that acupuncture is appropriate for all patients or conditions. However, there are many situations in which it is highly effective. By the simple procedure of inserting an acupuncture needle into a patient at a precisely diagnosed location, I have often seen the patient's pain begin to disappear. The Chinese refer to this as the restoration of the flow of energy, or *chi*.

My success in balancing the use of medical acupuncture and allopathic medicine is best reflected by two very special patients. Each has provided me the satisfaction of knowing that, by integrating many philosophical approaches to medicine, I can be a more effective physician.

The first case is a 50-year-old female who had a lifetime history of chronic sinusitis headaches. She had been to numerous physicians, including those specializing in immunology, neurology, and otolaryngology. In the course of therapy, she received the range of the modern pharmacopeia with little or no success. Although many of her problems were seasonal, her socioeconomic situation dictated that there was not much she could do to change her environment. Within three sessions of acupuncture, this patient became pain-free and has been without headaches for nearly 5 years.

The second patient was a 39-year-old female who had developed reflex sympathetic dystrophy in one of her lower extremities. Again, this was a patient for whom all of the treatments of modern allopathic and osteopathic medicine had failed. When she came to our clinic, her leg below her knee was discolored, swollen, extremely painful to light touch, and cold. After much discussion and consultation with my colleagues at the Arizona Pain Institute, we felt a regimen of acupuncture was justified. Literally within 30 to 40 minutes, you could see the extremity turn pink, improve in color, and decrease in sensitivity to pain. Although we have been unable to eliminate the pain totally, we have been successful in reducing it to a tolerable level. Unfortunately, each treatment is effective only for a month and must be repeated. Despite that, she has restored her optimistic attitude toward living.

Because of these and other patients, I have begun to appreciate that one's health not only involves scientifically demonstrated mechanisms but also a spiritual attitude of well-being and the wholeness of life. We as physicians must continue to pursue and integrate new philosophies into our medical armamentarium.

According to a landmark article, one in three adults used at least one form of alternative therapy in 1990. This would equate to about $14 billion of annual expenditure in the United States alone (Eisenberg et al., 1993). A recent nine-country European study identified patient utilization rates between 18% and 75% for alternative therapies. This growth in diversity of health care has been facilitated by legal recognition through licensing and certification of different kinds of alternative practitioners in many states (discussed in chapter 4) and through reimbursement mechanisms by third party payers (discussed in chapter 6). Through state legislation and/or insurance company policy, it is becoming commonplace for managed care plans to either capitate or provide risk contracts for alternative providers, such as chiropractors.

Growing research in alternative therapies also has propelled the reemergence of alternative medicine. Not only are new journals devoted to such research, but articles and guidelines have been published in recent years in mainstream scientific journals. Because of the strength of public interest, the National Institutes of Health (NIH) Office of Alternative Medicine was established in 1992 (Jacobs, 1995).

Biomedicine has been shown to be quite effective in the treatment of infectious diseases with antibiotics and in the management of acute trauma. But it has been estimated that conventional care may be the most appropriate and effective type of treatment for only 20% of the problems brought by patients to their conventional health care providers. In an age of cost containment and growing litigious concern over adverse outcomes, further questions have arisen about the significant costs and side effects of conventional therapies, medications, and technologies.

Other reasons for the reemergence of interest within medical education is the value of reintroducing alternative modalities to enhance the cultural sensitivity of students, increasingly important for preparing physicians to practice in multicultural and multiethnic settings. Improving the interview skills of physicians-in-training and thus enhancing the doctor-patient relationship and trust should be a major outcome of this enhanced training. When one considers that 72% of patients who see alternative practitioners do not reveal these visits to their mainstream physicians, a potentially volatile "dual parallel universe" of health care delivery systems exists in the United States.

Globally, it has been estimated that from 70% to 90% of all medical problems and episodes requiring some level of responsive care are dealt with in sites other than a Western-trained physician's office. Most often, medical problems are cared for in the home or within the folk or popular culture sector. In economically developing countries and areas of the United States (Native American reservations, economically depressed areas, and enclaves of recent immigrants), there has routinely been a strong emphasis on traditional healers and folk remedies. Though there have been successful integrative models developed in medical education in other parts of the world (Africa, China, India, Taiwan), Western medical education's efforts at integration have been more commonplace in Germany, France, and Sweden than in the United States. Nevertheless, using alternative therapy in the biomedical curriculum is beginning to emerge as a "bridge" toward more culturally sensitive training.

Since 1990 the Medical College of Pennsylvania has introduced to second-year medical students the role of folk and popular healing systems. Their goal is to improve the students' ability to recognize and work effectively with the lay beliefs and practices of their patients. It is the faculty's belief that the diverse cultural orientations that medical students will see in clinical practice will mandate their exposure to a variety of alternative therapies. A third-year special exam, the OSCE (Objective Standardized Clinical Examination), actually assesses and reinforces the student's abilities and skills at integrating the patient's health-beliefs history and arriving at a negotiated treatment plan.

These are essential building-block skills, leading toward a true integrative or complementary medicine paradigm, again based on initial objectives of broadening the cultural or ethnosensitivity of students. To keep pace with an increasingly multicultural society, Australian medical education is mainstreaming culturally appropriate ways to assure that graduates can effectively practice with patients of any cultural background, providing new courses in transcultural medicine and medical anthropology.

Currently, at least 34 medical schools in the United States have started or are developing courses focusing on alternative medical practices in their curriculum for the MD degree. Updated lists of courses on alternative therapies taught at conventional United States medical schools are available on the Internet (see "Representative Internet World Wide Web Sites," at the end of this chapter).

MEDICAL STUDENTS AS CHANGE AGENTS

The natural history of establishing new courses in medical schools covering alternative or complementary medicine topics begins most often with student interest. For instance, at the University of Arizona, health professions students (medical, nursing, and pharmacy) began meeting off-campus one evening every week in the early 1980s to explore with faculty facilitators the theory and practice of various alternative therapies. Eventually, strong attendance at these extracurricular offerings led to guest lectures in required courses and ultimately in electives; then structured, more formal curricula and courses evolved for the preclinical years. Ultimately, fourth-year electives were created for students to work in community settings with nonallopathic providers.

The response of the traditional medical faculty to these experimental courses in alternative medicine is mixed. However, various other approaches to broadening the traditional medical curriculum are evolving throughout the country. At Columbia University a grant helped establish a center for complementary medicine (see also chapters 12 and 13). The center's threefold goals have been to (1) coordinate and conduct rigorous scientific research on alternative and complementary medical therapies; (2) provide professional education to health care providers, medical students, and students at Columbia's schools of medicine, nursing, public health, and dentistry; and (3) be an authoritative source of information about alternative medicine for the general public and health care professions.

With limited resources, the center's first effort was to survey existing faculty with clinical and research expertise in nonstandard medical treatments. Next, a scientific advisory board composed of basic and clinical researchers was established. Collaborations were developed between departments, leading eventually to formal studies.

A number of professional societies, such as the Society of Teachers of Family Medicine (STFM), have developed working groups and a model curriculum by sharing their evolving approaches in medical schools around the country. Many medical schools are also offering continuing medical education courses to physicians. The University of Arizona's new Program in Integrative Medicine offers courses throughout the year covering botanical medicine, Chinese herbal medicine, tai chi, and other alternative therapies.

BASICS OF ALTERNATIVE THERAPY
MEDICAL EDUCATION PROGRAMS

Learner-centered curricula for medical students are appropriate for American medical schools where there is a shortage of faculty with experience in alternative medicine (Hansen, 1991). These curricular *objectives* can be achieved by students:

1. Knowledge about alternative therapies and the placebo effect, from both a scientific and a social point of view.
2. Skills in collaborative problem solving, including hypothesis formation and testing, to articulate ideas and arguments for one form of alternative diagnosis and treatment over another.
3. Attitudes of open-mindedness about patient autonomy and decision making and acceptance of alternative patient perspectives and health beliefs.

A proposed *curriculum* could include the following basic activities:

1. Pairs of students are randomly assigned one of various types of alternative therapies being practiced in their community and then are attached to a practitioner who has volunteered to become a community adjunct faculty member.

2. Students do a literature search on their alternative therapy, select and read key articles, and provide a summary to peers. Students determine what is considered to be the scientific basis for the therapy and describe ethical problems that they think might be encountered in its practice.

3. Students interview their community alternative practitioner and patients who have benefited from that alternative treatment, as well as dissatisfied patients, mainstream physicians, and relevant scientists, to assess whether the students' ideas as developed from literature review and observation are accurate.

4. Each student pair prepares arguments for and against the use of the particular form of alternative therapy as if to convince an educated, intelligent patient.

5. A half-day is allocated to students debating issues that have emerged during literature and field research.

6. The medical school faculty solicits the volunteer practitioners to become community adjunct faculty, formulates and explains the objectives and organization of the curriculum to the students and adjunct faculty, and acts as advisors to students throughout their literature and field research.

In summary, medical schools should develop objectives and curricula that are learner-centered. Such courses or programs could draw on community expertise, given the typical dearth of experienced faculty in alternative therapies.

IMPACT OF MANAGED CARE

With health care reform and the spread of managed care in the marketplace, new opportunities are emerging for the availability and integration of certain alternative therapies. This growing interest is stimulated by patient and payer demand to provide maximal value through enhancing quality and controlling cost. There is measurable "marketing value" (given that most potential customers already pay out-of-pocket for alternative forms of care) in making alternative therapies available. Some managed care organizations also feel that costs can be better managed (e.g., chiropractic care for low back pain rather than referral to an orthopedic surgeon). Although managed care is cost-driven, it also should be responsive to what purchasers want from health care delivery systems. The more common alternative services provided through managed care arrangements include chiropractic and diet and nutrition counseling programs. Usually, a plan's policy committee determines what kind of practitioners will be included.

Because the training of medical students and residents through academic medical centers and community-based settings is becoming increasingly dependent on managed care contracts, the policies established by managed care organizations will in many ways dictate the kinds of practice setting exposures and interactions students and residents will have with alternative providers. Ironically, a common experience for students and residents is dealing with the dissatisfied patient who is denied access to a certain form of alternative therapy not approved by the plan or is prevented by plan policy from seeing an approved alternative practitioner beyond a maximum number of visits.

The intended, prescribed goal of managed care is to deliver affordable, accessible, and quality health care, so it is quite likely that access to those approved alternative therapies that have proved cost-effective will expand in the years ahead. This broader coverage will likely be sensitive to and dependent on successful research outcomes in studies currently funded by the NIH Office of Alternative Medicine (OAM) and various other foundations that are comparing biomedical with alternative treatments. Indeed, the economic force behind managed care and consolidation in the health care industry may become the primary driving force for complementary medicine in the United States. One innovative health care company, American Western Life Insurance Company in Foster City, California, provides a panel made up only of alternative and wellness-oriented providers. Its health care plan and products are meant to complement biomedical health care.

Enrollment of insured persons starts with a lifestyle visit to a "wellness doctor" (a naturopathic physician), who reviews not just current conditions and symptoms but also reviews health goals, exercise, and environmental issues. Working with the patient, the doctor formulates an action plan for maintaining health. If a patient develops symptoms of disease, he or she can talk to a wellness doctor with access to the patient's wellness information file, who will guide the patient to a treatment plan or refer the patient to an appropriate care provider, beginning with the least invasive approach.

The openness of managed care plans and IPAs (for managed care abbreviations and definitions, see Table 6.2) to alternative providers is also affected by state legislative efforts to enact "any willing provider" laws, which allow any appropriately licensed provider to participate in managed care. Such bills are usually directed toward chiropractic and acupuncture and stipulate that a provider does not have to be an MD or DO to participate and receive reimbursement. Some feel that such laws are quite controversial because they supersede the fundamental role of the primary care physician as care manager.

To participate in these IPAs or other managed care arrangements, alternative providers are typically required to meet certain criteria: a valid license to practice a specific form of alternative care, with no outstanding complaints; malpractice insurance; access to peer review; and the ability to write medical reports.

Partnerships between academic medical centers and managed care organizations for the purpose of conducting collaborative research is promising. Typical research projects could include developing clinical protocols for integrating alternative therapies and outcome studies comparing conventional and nonconventional treatments for common problems.

For a list of resources on managed care coverage of alternative therapies, refer to the end of this chapter.

IMPACT OF TELECOMMUNICATION AND THE INTERNET

With revolutionary speed, medical education has been significantly affected by the growth of the Internet and telemedicine linkages since the early 1990s. Alternative providers and therapies have not been strangers to this new technology and thus are becoming increasingly interactive with medical educators and learners as well as the lay public.

In addition to numerous World Wide Web pages from various medical schools and with the NIH OAM providing information on alternative medicine, international listservers have cropped up for practitioners, mostly allopathic and osteopathic, to share their practice experience with alternative forms of therapy. This rapid spread of information is becoming a routine modality for learning new scientific knowledge and breakthroughs and is superseding the slower dissemination of original and applied research through journals, newsletters, and textbooks. A compendium of Internet self-care support groups and alternative health approaches of interest to patients and health professions alike is available (Ferguson, 1996; see also the end of this chapter for "Representative Internet World Wide Web Sites, Mailing Lists, Discussion Groups" in alternative therapies).

"Virtual" medical schools now exist across the planet and are likely to shape the further evolution of alternative and complementary medicine and to have an effect on mainstream practice patterns globally. Over a dozen medical journals and newsletters have developed in the 1990s as vehicles for health professionals to disseminate research findings and clinical practice models and guidelines.

GROWTH IN WORK FORCE OF ALTERNATIVE MEDICINE PRACTITIONERS

A significant increase in the supply of alternative medicine practitioners is anticipated over the next 13 years (Cooper & Stoflet, 1996). A recent study predicts that the supply of chiropractors, naturopaths, and practitioners of oriental medicine will grow by 88% by the year 2010, compared to a growth in the traditional physician supply of 16%. Major factors contributing to this increase are opening of new colleges training these practitioners; anticipated favorable regulatory legislation in a number of states, allowing licensure and certification; improvement in reimbursement secondary to "any willing provider" type of legislation, affecting both public and private insurers; and growth in public and professional acceptance of and interest in alternative medicine.

There are several implications of this growing complementary work force for traditional medical education in the United States. There could be increased interaction and communication between the physician and the alternative medicine practitioner and a resultant improvement in referring patients back and forth. Territorial issues and competitive economic conflicts also could proliferate. More traditional physicians, who do not want to lose potential revenue by referring to the complementary work force, could develop skills in alternative therapies through continuing medical education. With a growing number of alternative practitioners comes the need to adjust supply projections for the health professions work force and also the need to broaden the definition of medical education to include nonallopathic and nonosteopathic training programs.

IMPACT OF RESEARCH

The major development in promoting research on alternative therapies in recent years is the establishment in 1992 of the NIH OAM. Spearheaded by Senator Tom Harkin (D-Iowa) of the then Senate Labor–HHS–Education Appropriations Subcommittee, the OAM was initially set up to evaluate unconventional medical practices. Harkin (1995, p. 71) sees this office as having the potential to "build the bridges between conventional and traditional medicine, acknowledging the efficacy of certain therapies in the face of irrefutable proof, and putting the well-being of the patient foremost," and thereafter mainstreaming alternative practices. Implicit in the OAM "charter" is a realization that conventional research techniques are not always appropriate in the examination of alternative therapies. The effectiveness of various therapies cannot be determined by "breaking them down into a series of chemical reactions and physiological processes." This fundamental realization may lead to a broader scientific and evidence-based foundation for a more realistic theory on which we will need to enhance and reform our comprehensive medical education system. It has propelled the maturation of research interests in alternative complementary medicine throughout the nation's academic medical centers.

Most of the over $1 million in grant awards for 43 projects has been to academic medical centers throughout the country (see Table 14.1 for a representative list of institutions and research projects). These projects range from baseline studies of the prevalence of interest among patients and

TABLE 14.1   1993–1994 OAM Grant Awards

Modality	Condition	Institution
Acupuncture	Depression	U. of Arizona
Acupuncture	Osteoarthritis	U. of Maryland
Massage therapy	HIV infection	Morse Research Center
ElectrochemDCcurrent	Tumors	City of Hope Medical Center
Enzyme therapy	Mammary metastasis	American Health Fdn
Hypnosis	Chronic pain	Virginia Polytechnic Institute
Massage therapy	Postoperative outcomes	U. of Virginia
Chinese medicine	Premenstrual syndrome	Pacific College of Oriental Medicine
Antihepatitis plants	Treatment evaluation	Washington U.
Music therapy	Brain injury	Penn State U.
Energetic therapy	Basal cell cancer	Meninger Clinic
Hypnosis	Healing bone fractures	McLean Hospital
Homeopathy	Health	U. of California
Dance movement	Cystic fibrosis	Hahnemann U.
Chinese herbs	Common warts	Emory U.
Tai chi	Balance disorders	Northwestern U.
Guided imagery	Asthma	Lenox Hill Hospital
Imagery/immunity	Cancer/AIDS	George Washington U.
Support imagery	Breast cancer	U. of Texas
Manual palpation	Intervertebral motility	U. of Vermont
Chinese herbs	Hot flashes	Columbia U.
Macrobiotics	Cancer	U. of Minnesota
Acupuncture	Oral surgery postoperative pain	U. of Maryland
Ayurvedic	Parkinsonism	Southern Illinois U.
Biofeedback	Diabetes	Medical College of Ohio
Acumoxa	Breech version	Georgetown U.
Hypnotic imagery	Immune response to breast cancer	Good Samaritan Hospital of Oregon
Therapeutic touch	Immune response to stress	Medical U. of South Carolina
Antioxidants	Cancer	U. of Colorado

TABLE 14.1 *(Continued)*

Modality	Condition	Institution
Massage effects	HIV infection in babies	U. of Miami
Yoga	Heroin addiction	North Charles Mental Health Research and Training Foundation, Massachusetts
Yoga	Obsessive-compulsive disorder	Khalsa Foundation
Biofeedback	Pain	Fitzsimmons Army Medical Center
Ayurvedic	Health	Sharp Health Care
Chinese medicine	Chronic HIV infection	American College of TCM
Acupuncture	Hyperactivity	Virginia Commonwealth University
Massage	Bone marrow transplants	Dartmouth College
Intercessory prayer	Investigation	U. of New Mexico
EEG normalization treatment	Mild head trauma	Temple U.
Transcranial electrostimulation	Chronic pain	Baylor
Homeopathy	Mild brain injury	Spaulding Rehabilitation Hospital
Qi gong	Reflex sympathetic dystrophy	U. of Medicine and Dentistry, New Jersey

Adapted from *Alternative and Complementary Therapies* (October 1994, p. 20).

health practitioners and the study of referral patterns to comparing cost-effectiveness, efficacy, and clinical outcomes with various treatment modalities.

Establishment of the OAM has been an essential step to spearhead the acceptance of teaching alternative therapies in both undergraduate and graduate medical education courses and curricula. One of the key barriers to mainstreaming alternative medicine has been that many practitioners lacked critical research skills. With a cadre of researchers at the nation's most prestigious academic medical centers, alternative medicine will now follow the course of other traditional disciplines: extramural postdoctoral training, National Research Service Awards, and the Intramural Program for Clinical Fellows, among others.

In addition to the type of fellowship program at the University of Arizona, discussed below, the NIH will provide clinical fellows training in the conduct of field investigation and clinical trials of alternative therapies. The OAM has also stimulated the other institutes at NIH to provide awards to researchers in alternative medicine. In 1993 alone this provided almost $13 million of additional NIH support for alternative medicine research.

THE PRACTICE AND TEACHING OF ALTERNATIVE THERAPIES: MODELS FROM ARIZONA

Few models currently exist in which alternative therapies are mainstreamed into the delivery of routine health care most typically available to Americans throughout the country. One exemplary setting with integrated health care is the Arizona Center for Health and Medicine in Phoenix, Arizona. At the center, medical students and residents have the opportunity to observe and participate in a setting where patients have a choice and providers are knowledgeable about different types of treatments. The center provides primary care and is able to reach patients at their first point of contact to manage their care most effectively. Affiliated with the University of Arizona College of Medicine in Tucson, the center is a joint project of an integrated delivery system, Mercy Healthcare Arizona-Catholic Healthcare West. Its advisory board consists of insurance company executives as well as faculty from the College of Medicine.

The Arizona Center for Health and Medicine is a designated site not only for medical schools and residents but also for the new MD/DO fellowship training program in integrative medicine being established by the University of Arizona. In addition to clinical practice training, the center co-sponsors educational courses for health care providers on alternative paradigms in medicine and healing, homeopathy for primary care physicians, osteopathy and manual medicine for MDs, and mind-body-spirit medicine (Moore, 1995; see also chapter 6, this volume).

Routine medical services provided to patients include traditional Chinese medicine, acupuncture, homeopathy, nutritional therapy, Ayurvedic medicine, psychological counseling, Trager and Feldenkrais body awareness techniques, therapeutic massage, therapeutic touch, osteopathic manipulation, guided visual imagery, herbal therapy, and yoga and tai chi classes, in addition to aromatherapy, color, and dance and art therapies. Patients also are encouraged to do spiritual work as a standard part of every patient encounter.

The center participates in a number of managed care plans and, through capitated reimbursement schemes for primary care, is able to deliver care through the most cost-effective and appropriate therapeutic modality. Results have been high patient satisfaction and decreases in both emergency room and hospital utilization. Under the leadership of Andrew Weil, MD, the University of Arizona Health Sciences Center's Program of Integrative Medicine soon will be offering the nation's first 2-year fellowship program for board-certified physicians in family practice or internal medicine. The program's goal is eventually to develop a new board specialty and residency program in integrative medicine. Integrative (complementary) medicine has been defined as a discipline combining the best ideas and practices of biomedicine and alternative medicine, always keeping the best interest of the patient at heart. Rather than embrace unconventional medicine uncritically or reject conventional medicine, integrative medicine as a school of thought and approach to health care will identify and criticize unsound ideas and practices wherever they are found.

Planning for the fellowship curriculum began in December 1994 with the establishment of a national panel composed of experts in alternative modalities. The intent is to implement the results of this panel into the American College of Integrative Medicine. In addition to training a cadre of faculty that will eventually "seed" academic institutions throughout the country with similar programs in integrative medicine (teaching, research, and clinical care), the fellowship will provide two to four physicians a year as teachers of residents and medical students.

The curriculum for the fellowship will build on foundation courses in the philosophy of science and history of medicine, broadening the scope of both to include non-Western systems from other cultures, such as traditional Chinese medicine and Ayurvedic medicine. Emphases will be placed on mind-body medicine, spirituality in medicine, death and dying, the birth experience, and other critical aspects of health not sufficiently covered in the more traditional undergraduate and graduate medical education curriculum.

Core areas will include the basic ideas and theories of the major alternative systems of medicine and provide for practical experience with alternative practitioners. Fellows will receive in-depth training in a small number of alternative systems to master related methods. For instance, all fellows will be expected to master the technique of interactive guided imagery and two of the following three therapies: medical acupuncture, manual manipulation, and homeopathy. In addition to practical experience with alternative practitioner experts and key medical doctors who practice various alternative modalities, the fellowship will operate an Integrative Medicine Clinic as part of the University of Arizona health care system. Each fellow will be required to complete a research project and prepare a publishable manuscript on the related research. The clinic will provide the fellows with patients and a natural-setting laboratory to conduct practice-based research on clinical outcomes. In anticipation of the implementation of the fellowship, continuing medical education courses have begun for practicing physicians in the community.

CONCLUSION

Attitudes are changing, partially driven by economics, and biomedicine stands to lose a significant patient base as well as an opportunity to enhance the health status of the public. Research in academic medical centers, especially interdisciplinary efforts comparing biomedical and alternative therapies, must continue. At a minimum, we must continue to teach medical students and residents a broader awareness of alternative therapies so that they can effectively communicate with the majority of their patients who use such therapies routinely. Perhaps American medical education will evolve an integrative approach and mind-set. An effective model of integrating alternative with biomedical therapies could be through primary care practice. Thus, efforts at teaching alternative therapies in medical education should be closely linked with new curricular reform plans throughout the United States designed to enhance student and resident exposure and experience in general.

The role of educating health professionals in training and in the community will continue to evolve within our nation's academic and community-based medical centers. Physicians should know the resources and skills available in their alternative medical community and how best to counsel their patients objectively about the potential for both good and harm in certain techniques. As care managers, primary care physicians can direct patients toward alternative practitioners with a reasonable scope of practice related to the patient's health beliefs. Educating the public on how they can most safely access alternative therapies—to benefit from the integrative and complementary nature of the best in alternative and biomedicine—must be objective and ideally done as a joint endeavor involving both types of practitioners.

Integrative medicine is likely to become commonplace in our nation's evolving health care delivery system. As interdisciplinary teams become the dominant way to care for individuals and families, an integrative medicine specialist (a biomedical physician with fellowship training in integrative medicine) will become an important team member, assessing patients who may benefit from an alternative therapy. With health centers capitated for the care of patient populations, increasingly the cost-effectiveness and cost-benefit ratio of blending alternative therapies with biomedical care will be well studied and confirmed.

Whenever possible, the cognitive aspects of alternative therapies will likely be delivered in new ways through medicine's digitalized future: patients will receive long-distance medical diagnosis and treatment and routine care through electronic home visits. Ultimately, within perhaps 10 to 15 years, the distinctions between biomedicine and alternative therapy will evaporate, and health care providers will participate in a core holistic medical education curriculum, branching off to specialize in a particular modality or technical skill or remaining integrative specialists.

RESOURCES FOR FURTHER INFORMATION

REPRESENTATIVE COURSES ON ALTERNATIVE THERAPIES TAUGHT AT CONVENTIONAL U.S. MEDICAL SCHOOLS

Boston University School of Medicine, Boston, MA
    "Public Health Perspectives on Alt Health Care" Allan R. Meyers
       (617/638-5042)
Case Western Reserve School of Medicine, Cleveland, OH
    "Chinese Qigong," Tianyou Hao (216/368-2229)
Emory University School of Medicine, Atlanta, GA
    "Complementary Medical Practices," Linda R. Gooding, PhD
       (404/727-5948)
Georgetown University School of Medicine, Washington, DC
    "The Program of Mind-Body Studies," James S. Gordon, MD
       (202/966-7338)
Harvard Medical School, Boston, MA
    "Alt Medicine: Implications for Clinical Practice and Research,"
       David M. Eisenberg, MD (617/735-3995)
    "Medical Hypnosis and Behavioral Therapy," Owen Surman
       (617/726-2991)
Indiana University School of Medicine, Indianapolis, IN
    "Complementary Medicine, Developing New Health Paradigms,"
       Vimal Patel (317/274-4662)
Johns Hopkins School of Medicine, Baltimore, MD
    "The Philosophy and Practice of Healing," Gail Geller, ScD, and
       Robert M. Duggan, MAc (410/955-7894)
Mount Sinai School of Medicine, New York, NY
    "Survey Course in Alt Medicine," "The Power of Subtle Body:
    Innovative Qigong," "Mind-Body Techniques and Healing,"
       "Hypnotherapy," "Intro to Biofeedback Techniques and Medical
       Practice,"

"Preparation for Certification in Biofeedback," "Science of Yoga,"
    Joyce Shriver, PhD (212/241-7273)
Rush Medical College, Chicago, IL
    "Foundations in Holistic Health," Tamara Heberlein (303/449-2820)
Southern Illinois University School of Medicine, Springfield, IL
    "Chinese Acupuncture," "Comparative Systems of Healing,"
        Cris Milliken (217/782-6124)
Stanford University School of Medicine, Palo Alto, CA
    "Alt Medicine: Scientific Perspective," W. Sampson, MD
        (408/885-4146)
University of Arizona College of Medicine, Tucson, AZ
    "Alt Medicine," Andrew Weil, MD (520/647-7858)
University of California, Los Angeles School of Medicine, Los Angeles, CA
    "Psychoneuroimmunology," Fawzy I. Fawzy, MD (310/825-0249)
    "Medical Acupuncture for Physicians," Joseph Helms, MD
        (510/841-7600)
    "Intro to Complementary Medicine," David Diehl, MD (818/364-3205)
    "Integrative East West Medicine," Ka Kit Hui, MD (310/206-1895)
University of California, San Francisco School of Medicine,
    San Francisco, CA
    "The Healer's Art," Rachel Naomi Remen, MD (415/868-2642)
    "Intro to Homeopathic Medicine," Michael Carlston, MD
        (707/545-1554)
    "Complementary Ways of Healing," Ellen Hughes, MD
        (415/476-3185)
University of Iowa, Iowa City, IA
    "Intro to Integrative Medicine" series, Evan Kligman, MD
        (319/335-8454)
University of Louisville School of Medicine, Louisville, KY
    "Alt and Paranormal Health Claims," Thomas Wheeler (502/852-6287)
University of Virginia School of Medicine, Charlottesville, VA
    "Healing Options: Complementary Medicine for Physicians of the
        Future," Pali Delevitt (804/924-2094)
Yale School of Medicine, New Haven, CT
    "Alt Medicine in Historical Perspective" Maria Trumpler
        (203/785-4338)
    "The Mind and Medicine," Howard P. Kahn, PhD (203/624-9411)

A complete list has been compiled by AMR'TA (Alchemical Medicine
Research and Teaching Association), with input from Office of Alternative
Medicine, NIH; Rosenthal Center for Alternative/Complementary Medicine,
Columbia University; and members of the Paracelsus Internet mailing list.

Programs can be viewed at http://www.teleport.com:80/~amrta or added by e-mail: amrta@amrta.org.

REPRESENTATIVE INTERNET WORLD WIDE WEB SITES,
MAILING LISTS, DISCUSSION GROUPS

Acupuncture: http://www.acupuncture.com/
    http://www.demon.co.uk/acupuncture/index.html
Alexander Technique: http://www.life.uiuc.edu/jeff/alextech.html
Algy's Herb Page: http://frank.mtsu.edu/~sward/herb.html
Alt Medical Resources (U of Pitt): http://www.pitt.edu/~cbw/altm.html
Alt Medicine Research: e-mail: majordomo@virginia.edu
AANP (Am Assoc of Nat Physicians):
    infinity.dorsai.org/naturopathic.physician
AMR'TA (discussion groups, mailing lists): e-mail: amrta@amrta.org
Ayurvedic Foundation: http://www.ayur.com
Chiropractic: http://www.mbnet.mb.ca/~jwiens/chiro.html
    http://www.syspac.com/~ezikmun
    http://www.amerchiro.org/aca
Cranial Osteopathy: http://www.users.dircon.co.uk/~med-man
Gen Council/Register Nat: http://www.compulink.co.uk/~naturopa-
    thy/welcome.htm
HERB list, Medicinal & Aromatic Plans: e-mail:
    LISTSERV@VM3090.EGE.EDU.TR
Herb Research Foundation: http://www.crl.com/~robbee/herbal.html
Homeopathy: http://www.dungeon.com/-cam/homeo.html
    http://community.net/-neils/faqhom.html
    wolfenet.com/-enos/ho-web/index.html
    http://antenna.nl/homeoweb
Nat Med, Compl Health Care, Alt Therapies:
    http://www.amrta.org/~amrta
OrMed (Oriental Medicine): //ftp.cts.com/pub/nkraft/ormed.html
Osteopathic Medicine:
    http://.www.demon.co.uk/osteopath/index.html
    http://www.rscom.com/osteo
Reiki and Reiki: http://www.skagit.com/turtle/reiki/ (and)
    http://www.crl.com/~davidh/reiki
Rosenthal Center for Alt/Complementary Medicine (Columbia
    University): http://cpmcnet.columbia.edu/dept/rosenthal/
Scientific Research on the Transcendental Meditation Program:
    http://www.mum.edu/TM_Research/TM_research_home.html
Shaman: e-mail: listserv@lisstserv.aol.com

http://www.webcom.com/gspirit/Shaman/shamanov.html
http://www.webcom.com/gspirit/Shaman/Usenet/srs.faq.html
USDA Herbal info (James Duke): http://www.ars-grin.gov/~ngrlsb/

RESOURCES FOR FURTHER INFORMATION ON MANAGED CARE COVERAGE OF ALTERNATIVE THERAPIES

American Association of Health Plans (AAHP) 202-778-3249
   (created in 1996 by the merger of American Managed Care and Review
    Association and Group Health Insurance)
American Western Life Company 415-573-8041
California Acupuncture Association 619-270-1005
Clinical Partners Health Resource Center 415-487-2800

15

Alternative Therapies: Quo Vadis?

Rena J. Gordon

*Synergistic: A remedy acting similarly to another remedy
and increasing its efficiency when combined with it.*
—*Edmund Ray Long, AB, MD, PhD*

As the United States health care system has grown in size and complexity over the past three decades, so too has consumer disillusionment with aspects of the biomedical system. Not only are delivery systems poorly coordinated, leaving patients to negotiate a complex maze of providers and services, but many diseases and health problems continue to burden the health care system and public health agencies. Costs of health care have continued to rise, and an increasing proportion of Americans either lack health insurance completely or have insufficient coverage.

Americans have sought relief from this system and explored a general state of wellness by turning to alternative therapies and practitioners and to the natural foods and products associated with alternative medicine. Alternative therapies satisfy consumer desire for cost control and for information and empowerment. The purpose of this book has been to provide a framework for understanding terms and concepts associated with alternative therapies and a forum for an interdisciplinary discussion of salient issues. It is designed to be useful to the newcomer to the field and to provide new insights to those familiar with alternative medicine.

Throughout the book run a number of common themes and consistent findings. Themes show either tendencies that push toward complementarity in medicine or constraints that pull away from achieving complementarity. Six key themes reveal that alternative medicine is (1) propelled by consumer interest, (2) associated with demographic characteristics of the population, (3) reflected in spatial distributions, (4) facing dilemmas about becoming professionalized or legitimized, (5) affected by characteristics of the American scientific community, and (6) driven by the engine of economics.

THE CONSUMER QUEST FOR WELLNESS

Physician Andrew Weil (1996) spoke of the tremendous potential in reversing chronic disease through a change in lifestyle, emphasizing that nutrition is a central element of a healthy lifestyle. As part of that lifestyle change, more people are demanding produce that is free of pesticides, herbicides, growth hormones, waxes, and fungicides. Produce that carries the heaviest toxic load currently includes strawberries, bell peppers, spinach, United States-grown cherries, peaches, Mexican-grown cantaloupe, celery, apples, apricots, green beans, grapes from Chile, and cucumbers. The Environmental Working Group claims that reducing consumption of these 12 foods, called the "dirty dozen," can cut health risk from pesticides in produce by 50% (Weil, 1996).

In California, support of organic agriculture is entirely in response to consumer pressure. Successful demand in that state has resulted in a high rate of conversion to large-scale organic agriculture, making pesticide-free produce widely available at reasonable prices in many areas of the state. Although demand is present elsewhere, other states have not yet caught up to California in large-scale organic agriculture. This limits the availability and variety of organic produce in most American communities and increases the costs. The California example indicates how consumers can have a major influence in securing pesticide-free produce as part of emergent health concerns.

The power of consumers to effect change is revealed in several chapters. The first example showing grass-roots effectiveness comes from chapter 3, regarding the repeal of the Nutritional Labeling Enforcement Act (NLEA). The FDA had supported the NLEA because it gave them great regulatory authority to enforce prohibitions against the sale of vitamins and supplements. A groundswell of public opinion led to the repeal of the NLEA and the substitution of the Dietary Supplement Health Education Act (DSHEA). With the passage of the latter, the FDA suffered a loss of power over alternative medicine, because FDA enforcement efforts to curtail the marketing of nutriceuticals were halted.

A second example of the strength of consumer action is found in chapter 4, which examined the role of the state in respect to licensure and legitimation. In many states without provider practice acts, alternative practitioners can still practice. The case of North Carolina is an example where strong lobbying from supporters of alternative health care made homeopathy and nonmedical acupuncture legal (chapters 4 and 5). The power of the state aside, health professions can grow or wither on their own merit or misfortune by word-of-mouth recommendations or vilification from patients.

A third example concerns insurance coverage of alternative therapies, noted in chapter 6. A case was given of Blue Cross of Washington and Alaska, which decided to offer coverage of alternatives after customers bombarded the company with that request. Customers also are contacting their employers' benefits personnel or going directly to their insurers to remind them that their competitors are starting to offer this coverage. Consumer requests are meeting with success because more companies are providing coverage by reimbursing for selected alternative practices. This success also can reflect, in part, cost savings to insurance companies for less expensive alternative treatments.

A fourth example is found in chapter 7. Alternative practitioners usually locate their practice where there is demand from clients or patients. The pattern for three western states noted that demand is greatest (reflected in high provider-to-population ratios) in secondary, nonmetropolitan areas of high income levels and in areas of high amenities.

A fifth example of consumer-driven response, the case of childbirth, is discussed in chapter 8. Over the past few decades, some women and a few physicians began to question the assumption that pregnancy and childbirth always required medical management and intervention. The women's movement encouraged women to demand control of their childbearing decisions, and many decided that most home birth and midwife-attended births were both safe and preferable. Women have gained more choices in birthing, and midwives have become increasingly mainstream, co-opted by the biomedical establishment.

A sixth example, mentioned in a number of chapters, is the NIH Office of Alternative Medicine created by Congressional mandate. The development of this office represents the effects of consumer demand of their political representatives to provide an officially sanctioned clearinghouse of information, as well as to conduct research on efficacy of alternative practices.

A seventh example of grass-roots success appears in chapter 14, which discusses how medical students act as change agents of the medical curricula. An example from the University of Arizona is given. In the next section, on demographic trends, an amplification of consumer demand is discussed in relation to the size and characteristics of the baby boom cohort.

DEMOGRAPHIC CHARACTERISTICS

One thing is certain: the growing demand for alternative therapies is consumer-driven. Alternative therapies are meeting a need not satisfied by biomedicine. Demographically, America is aging, and the health needs of an aging population provide a growing market for health care. According to the United States Bureau of the Census (1996b), of the 76 million baby boomers in the United States one will be hitting age 50 every 7.5 seconds for the next 15 years. By 2030, 20% of the country's population is expected to be 65 or older. This age cohort is so large that it has always driven the market for goods and services, and its sheer size dominates the demographic landscape.

Analyst Cheryl Russell (1993), in her thesis that the baby boom generation is remaking America, also notes that this generation of aging Americans differs from those that preceded it. They are well traveled and the most highly educated generation in American history. As youths they backpacked the world, experiencing other cultures and societies. This firsthand exposure makes them more open to cross-cultural ideas about health and healing than less-traveled past generations. Also, advances in worldwide computer communication networks make the baby boomers the most globally aware generation.

They also are more individualistic, believing that the self-interest of the individual supersedes the shared interest of the community. The belief in the primacy of the individual finds them "obsessed with their own bodies" (Russell, 1993, p. 164). They will form enormous markets for products and services that promise to stop or slow the aging process. Millions of baby boomers now belong to local health clubs and are turning to antiaging remedies, including natural foods, herbs, and vitamins. Other evidence of trying to turn back the hands of time is the growing use of cosmetic surgery. The first liposuction was performed in the United States in 1982, and by 1992 about 112,000 were performed annually (Russell, 1993).

As Russell notes, baby boomers tend to be spiritual in a different way than the previous generation. Spirituality, as defined by them, is a private expression of faith rather than an institutionalized religious faith. Their spiritual quest is a renewed search for the meaning of life. Spiritual therapies fall right into their belief structure. Medical pluralism, or accepting differing healing systems, presents fewer problems for baby boomers than for previous generations. For example, the model of complementary medicine presented in chapter 2, which categorizes alternative therapies as body healing, mind-spirit, and cross-cultural, falls within the understanding and experience of baby boomers.

Meredith McGuire (1988) supports the idea that this "new class" of baby boomers is bringing about change with respect to a middle-class healing movement. Although alternative therapies are not new, McGuire notes, the new class (baby boom cohort) is well placed at this point in history to produce change. This group is more educated and more articulate than others. "Often ideas and practices that have been present in previous historical periods become significant or potent in a period when they are linked with an ascendent or socially effective group" (p. 256).

The American population is getting older, as a result of the aging baby boom cohort. It is also becoming more culturally and ethnically diverse. Diversity suggests growing acceptance of medical pluralism. The percentage of the total U.S. population in 1996 (265,253,000) that is White (excluding Hispanic, which is included in non-White) is 73. This is projected to shrink to 70% of the total in 2010 and to 52.7% in 2050 (U.S. Bureau of the Census, 1996a, Table 1). By the year 2056, the U.S. census projects an even split in the percentage of White and non-White populations.

Examples from chapters in the book speak to this growing trend, including the shamanistic healing practices of different ethnic groups in the United States, described in chapter 9. Each household in America possesses a rich repository of health beliefs and practices that illustrate the ethnic origins and history of the household members. Examples of household medical systems in the hill country of Texas reflect residents' German heritage in healing beliefs and practices and are presented in chapter 10. Relationships in the healing process differ by culture. From an example of *Espiritismo*, as practiced in Puerto Rico and in other areas of Latin America, the healer-client relationship is analyzed in chapter 11. American medical schools are sensitizing students to the reality that they will be serving an increasing number of patients from multicultural backgrounds. Alternative medicine has emerged as an important new curricular component in over 30 mainstream medical schools and is described in chapter 14.

SPATIAL PATTERNS

Locational aspects of alternative medicine are investigated in several chapters. Because it is known that innovations do not diffuse uniformly over space, observing where alternative therapies are clustered provides an understanding of the spread of the phenomenon (Meade, Florin, & Gesler, 1988, p. 313).

Data aggregated by state and/or region (in chapters 4–6, 8, and 13) showed striking patterns. A bicoastal pattern was revealed in statutes for the practice of acupuncture, enrollment in HMOs, midwife-assisted deliveries, and membership in the American Holistic Medical Association (AHMA). The same general spatial pattern is displayed on diverse factors.

For example, states with acupuncture practice acts are generally located adjacent to the Pacific and Atlantic coasts and (one state) bordering the Gulf of Mexico. Statutes were passed earliest (1970–1979) in states along the Pacific Coast and the Gulf of Mexico, as well as in some western Mountain states. The midwestern, or heartland, states have no statutes.

Participation in managed care varies across the country. States with the highest enrollment in HMOs suggest a regional pattern, with highest enrollment on the Pacific Coast, the Southwest, and the north and mid-Atlantic coast. America's heartland has the lowest enrollment.

Of the percentage of births attended by midwives in 1990, the largest occurred in the New England, South Atlantic, Mountain, and Pacific Coast states. The smallest percentage occurred in the Midwest.

Using U.S. census regions, the highest proportion of physicians who were members of the AHMA was found in the West. Also, a general comment in chapter 5, on homeopathy, indicated that residents in northern and western states were especially attracted to homeopathic medicine. There are three United States colleges (see chapters 4 and 6) offering degrees in naturopathic medicine, all of which are in the West (Arizona, Oregon, and Washington).

Innovation on the coasts, especially on the West Coast, is not new to American society. Some time ago, the historian Frederick Jackson Turner noted about the western frontier: "This expansion westward with its new opportunities . . . furnish the forces dominating American character" (Wish, 1960, p. 190).

Studies on the diffusion of innovation (Brown, 1968; Hagerstrand, 1968) support the findings that new ideas gain a foothold in areas where people are exposed to the exchange of ideas, whether from other cultures, as in coastal areas, or from formal educational institutions, such as university towns.

In an example from a study on religion it was noted that, "befitting their geographic location at the center of the country, Midwesterners provide a remarkably true reflection of most measures of religion in America" (Gallup & Bezilla, 1996, p. F15). Thus, a measure of the success of an innovation is whether it diffuses to and eventually takes hold in the heartland. Whether this will occur for the practice of alternative medicine remains to be seen.

THE DILEMMA OF LEGITIMATION AND OTHER DICHOTOMIES

At the interface of alternative practices with biomedicine and within alternative medicine itself, dichotomies surface. The dilemma for many alternative practitioners is whether becoming legitimized and gaining respectability is worth the cost to their independence of practice. As discussed in chapters 4 and 6, legitimation to practice alternative medicine is affected by many factors. Although legitimation encompasses a broad range of factors, state laws and policies play a decisive role in stature, acceptance, and professionalization (Abbott, 1988). State licensure and/or registration are important, but as noted in chapter 4, legitimation to practice alternative medicine can exist independently of state sanction.

Public legitimation also can be influenced by word of mouth, professional competition, news coverage, personalities of individual providers, and the familiarity of a health care setting. Studies being conducted at NIH and elsewhere on the efficacy of alternative medicine will affect legitimation, either to enhance or to diminish specific therapies, depending on study results.

The inclusion of alternative health care in formulating health policy, coupled with freedom from physician oversight, could increase the standing of alternative providers as accepted health professionals. Reimbursement by insurance companies and inclusion in managed care plans serve as other components of legitimation. With all these factors operating toward legitimation, some alternative providers fear that the result might be a two-edged sword.

An example of this dilemma is found in chapter 6, which notes that many alternative providers in Washington State view the law passed January 1, 1996, with dual feelings. The law mandates that health insurance companies cover any licensed provider, which includes alternative therapists licensed in the state. This law is likely to result in a significant increase in consumers' access to alternative therapies, but because the services will be covered by indemnity insurance and managed care plans, the incorporation of insurance payments into a medical practice brings with it a whole array of additional complications. These complications include requirements for payment by insurers, such as use of specific billing forms, coding, and possible prior authorization of services. Billing clerks have to be hired, and the practice no longer operates on a simple cash basis. Life suddenly becomes more complicated for alternative health care providers as they join the economic mainstream and the corporatization of American health care. Some alternative providers fear that the process of legitimation spins a diverting web not worth the entanglement.

The dilemma of power in the physician-patient relationship is examined in chapters 10 and 11. In a relationship where the physician has power to make clinical and other decisions for a patient or has control over resources, power both constrains and enables. Patients, when asked, do not always want more control over their treatment. They hold trust in their physician as the most important component of their relationship. Yet, as Koss-Chioino notes, control over resources can lead to domination as well as to exploitation in matters of health and illness. Relationship with a physician-healer can be appreciated as a two-edged sword for a patient. Caring, curing, and relief are the benefits of trust and authority, but the price might be domination over life decisions, disease definition, and values.

In chapter 3 the dichotomy in the political arena is evident in the controversies over the role of the federal FDA. There is the collective responsibility of the government to eliminate fraudulent treatments. Federal laws are designed to protect the consumer against potential harm from unsafe and ineffective health products in the marketplace. To enforce these laws, Congress delegated broad regulatory power to several federal agencies; perhaps the most powerful, for both alternative and biomedicine, is the FDA. Some of their enforcement efforts have been singled out as the most egregious examples of government suppression of medical freedoms; critics of the agency cite their blatant ties to the pharmaceutical industry and their arbitrary regulation of nutritional supplements and herbs.

Does this agency act as a protector of the public's health or as a protector of established biomedical financial interests that limit individual freedoms in the choice of medical care? Although the controversy still exists, with strong forces operating on either side, the decision regarding supplements has weakened the power of the FDA in relation to alternative medicine.

The dichotomies experienced by alternative providers as they become more legitimatized, by patients as they put power in the hands of physicians-healers, and by the federal government as it defines its role as a protector of the public's health lead to another dichotomy mentioned in many chapters, the mind-body dualism of biomedicine. Also referred to as a reductionist model, biomedicine has traditionally limited its focus to the material, or body, and has left the mind to others, historically to religion. This dualism is at the heart of a raging debate in science, one that affects how alternative therapies are viewed by the biomedical community as well as by consumers.

CHARACTERISTICS OF THE AMERICAN SCIENTIFIC COMMUNITY

Healing and religion have been tightly integrated throughout most of history. One characteristic of modern Western biomedicine is that the mind and body have been separated. It is a false dichotomy, according to neuroscientist Candace Pert (1995), whose discoveries of peptide receptors led to an understanding of the chemicals that travel between the mind and the body. The notion that the mind is somehow distinct from the body goes back to an agreement that Descartes was forced to make with the Roman

Catholic Church. Descartes was allowed to study science, as we know it, if he "left the soul, the mind, the emotions, and consciousness to the realm of the church" (Pert, 1995, pp. 179–180). Western science has come a long way with that reductionist paradigm, but increasingly things do not quite fit into it. Much of what we are dealing with now may have to do with the integration of mind and matter.

Evidence of the integration is found in examples throughout this book. Discussed in chapter 12 are differences between "doing" and "being" nursing therapies. An example from the latter category is guided imagery. "Being" therapies are based on theories ranging from spiritual, metaphysical, and psychological to new physiological understandings. Listed in chapter 9 are shamanistic healing beliefs and practices among racial and ethnic groups in America, as, for example, *curanderismo,* which holds to belief in the inseparability of mind and body. Given in chapter 10 are examples of how some Texas hill country residents still incorporate faith healing and other alternative practices within their household medical systems. Discussed in chapter 11 are healing relationships in *Espiritismo,* a shamanistic healing process in Puerto Rico and other parts of Latin America. The literature, as well as clinical evidence from the success of Dean Ornish's treatment program (which includes meditation to prevent and reverse the ravages of heart disease), suggests the important role of the mind, consciousness, spirituality, and emotions in healing. Because the best practitioners treat the whole person, not just the physical manifestation of the disease or symptom, they often explore the links in the mind-body connection. Considered in chapter 13 are physicians who practice holistic medicine.

There is a growing body of literature, much of it European, indicating that emotional history is extremely important in illness. For example, it appears that suppression of grief and of anger, in particular, are associated with an increased incidence of breast cancer in women. Some argue that, on the mind-body schism, the biomedical community has taken on the role the Catholic Church held earlier (Pert, 1995). The negative effects of dominance of either side of the mind-body debate indicate that

> [a]s long as the debate hinges on the issue of dominance, both sides will fail
> . . . domination of one part of ourselves over all the other parts is an archaic,
> improper, and indefensible concept. For matter does not dominate mind, nor
> does mind dominate the body. (Dossey, 1984, p. 113)

Critics of alternative medicine say alternative medical treatments have not passed enough clinical trials to show efficacy. Some physicians are concerned that people with serious illnesses will reject standard treatments in favor of alternative therapies that have not worked. Proponents of alternative therapies counter with the fact that a great many things in standard medicine are not proven either, but physicians do them nevertheless. Alternative medicine "represents the rediscovery of a different way of thinking about health, one that forsakes rigid medical models and looks instead to natural ways of helping the body to heal itself" (Weil, cited in Kolata, 1996a, p. C1).

How can these divergent views find some common ground? A first attempt may be to look at the notion of science. Science takes place in a social-cultural context (Kuhn, 1970). Topics that undergo scientific testing do so because science studies what society values.

> Certainly as a society, we have some choice in what research developments we choose to pursue more vigorously, how much we will invest, and where we wish to place our limited resources. These choices will be governed not [only] by the inherent logic of medical developments but rather by our definitions of what is important and what we value. (Mechanic, 1979, p. 175)

The historic division of body and mind is paralleled by a division of the material and spiritual world. Scientists are not comfortable in the spiritual realm because they have been trained to look at that realm as outside science. Therefore, science has not put effort, resources, or value into studying the realm of the mind in the mind-body connection. One can understand why there is criticism that alternative medicine generally is based on anecdotal rather than scientific evidence. A corollary of this argument would be to blame the victim. Science does not study alternative therapies concerning spirit or soul because they are unknowable and beyond their definition of scientific inquiry. Circular reasoning based on fear of the unknown or reluctance to change borders on dogma. There is overwhelming evidence that discoveries that do not fit into the existing paradigm are denied for years (Pert, 1995).

Other factors contribute to a lack of scientific evidence regarding the efficacy of alternative medicine. Securing resources for research is highly competitive. In a climate of increasingly constrained resources, diverting funds to alternative medical research at the expense of biomedical research is not welcome. Also, methodologies for studying alternative therapies must be developed because those that work for the body do not necessarily work for the mind. The current methods might cause problems for the scientist limited by the biomedical model. Central to current scientific investigations are the guidelines that the treatment must be applied to each patient in exactly the same way, to isolate its effects from other influences. According to Marvin Zelen, a statistician who specializes in clinical trial design, "you need a protocol where therapies are reproducible" (cited in Kolata, 1996b, p. B7).

Proponents of studying alternative therapies note that clinical trials are not always possible and may not be appropriate. Many therapies are individually tailored and often used by practitioners who follow no uniform method. Studies that insist on uniformity cannot capture the essence of the treatments, argues psychologist Thomas Kiresuk (cited in Kolata, 1996b, p. B7). Methods of energy manipulation systems, discussed in chapter 12, are used by some nurses to influence health. Scientists do not yet know how to represent this kind of energy. New methods and tools for studying this form of energy probably will be discovered by a physicist, someone outside medicine (Pert, 1995). A positive trend is that more branches of science are beginning to overlap and converge.

The paradoxes, the unexplainable, or the mystery of why something works present great opportunities for science. For example, "being" therapies of nursing fall into the paradoxical healing category because they frequently happen without an apparent scientific explanation. "A paradox is a seemingly absurd or contradictory statement or event that is, in fact, true" (Dossey et al., 1995, pp. 16–17). It is these very paradoxes, or anomalies, that are the most fruitful for scientific investigation. This is the way new advances are made in our understanding and could lead to new insights and new theories. How best will these new opportunities be operationalized? A team approach, the merging of research by drawing from the physical and social sciences, is the direction for the future.

THE ENGINE OF ECONOMICS

Alternative therapies, although varied and diverse in theory and practice, emphasize prevention of disease and maintaining good health. They often focus on stimulating the body's natural defenses rather than focus on attacking germs and bacteria. Educating people about lifestyle changes and self-care is an important aspect of disease prevention. Prevention has major cost-saving implications.

The concept of prevention of disease is not new. In Greek mythology the goddess of healing, Panacea, was a proponent of a remedy for all ills or difficulties, or a cure-all. The goddess of health, Hygeia, prescribed a moderate and balanced life. Healing versus prevention, as represented by these two mythological figures, has competed for dominance in health care over the centuries. Modern Western biomedicine embraced Panacea's concepts with drugs and costly high-tech interventions, overshadowing those of Hygeia, which prescribe prevention—holistic, noninvasive, less expensive, personalized medicine. Americans have had the widespread belief that for every problem of life there is a pill, a bottle of medicine, or another instant cure. The pendulum, however, has swung too far in the direction of incredibly expensive high-tech medicine that is bankrupting the country (Pert, 1995, pp. 191–192).

A change in this trend challenges the medical profession and the drug and equipment manufacturers, who have much to protect in dominance, prestige, and profit. The reality is that prevention saves money, and this idea is attracting interest in the marketplace of individuals, employers, insurance companies, and increasing numbers of health care professionals. The American Academy of Anti-Aging Medicine is a new medical specialty formed in 1993 by a dozen physicians and researchers. By 1997, membership in the Academy had grown to 1,500. Early detection, prevention, and reversal of age related disease is the approach of this new medical field (Klatz & Kahn, 1997). Prevention is having an impact on the manufacturing sector of the economy as well. For example, the medically documented negative health effects of smoking are being adjudicated in the courts, with large dollar settlements imposed on cigarette manufacturers. Because alternative therapies emphasize prevention, increasingly they are being included in strategies to lower health care costs.

The health care marketplace is highly competitive. Alternative medicine, like biomedicine, is becoming more aggressive in marketing and targeting certain audiences. As noted in chapter 6, biomedical providers have increasingly shifted from targeting consumers to insurance and managed care companies. Marketing channels for alternative providers continue to target consumers, who pay directly out of pocket for services. As more insurance and managed care companies reimburse for selected alternative therapies, their marketing channels will target both consumers and insurers. Competition, if not a monopoly, can be a positive factor in expanding choices at a lower cost.

Because most alternative therapies are still paid for directly by consumers, alternative practitioners may be locating in high-end markets, as noted in chapter 7. As insurance reimbursements become more common, this distributional pattern is likely to diffuse to lower-end markets.

Economic considerations also are major factors behind co-optations of alternative therapies by the biomedical establishment. Recent shifts to managed care and emphasis on the bottom line have resulted in a decrease in physician income. One strategy in the competition for patients is to co-opt ideas and practices from alternative medicine. With a decreasing number of births, competition for birthing services led obstetricians and hospitals to employ nurse-midwives and establish birthing centers to attract patients, as noted in chapter 8. Through changes in medical school curricula, new physicians are being trained to include alternative therapies in their awareness and future medical practice. An illustration of how an established physician can acquire skills in medical acupuncture is included in chapter 14.

The economic engine also operates for patients who try to receive the best care at the most reasonable cost. The household medical system devises a cost-effective strategy among choices in a pluralistic system, as suggested in chapter 10. An emphasis throughout this book is the importance of a pluralistic system in medicine. Monopolies in medicine, as in other sectors of the economy, are ultimately counterproductive to achieving the most effective health system.

Monopolies in any sector of the economy tend to become complacent. The United States auto industry, as an example, lost market share to Japan because it did not change to meet the demand for smaller, more efficient cars. After more than 20 years, Detroit made a comeback by finally producing reliable and efficient cars at prices comparable to those of their competitors.

In health care (a sector of the economy that consumes one seventh, or 14% of the Gross National Product), biomedicine has had a monopoly for over 70 years. Medical pluralism flourished in the United States in the 19th and early 20th centuries; and according to economic indicators alone, it is making a major comeback. As noted, Americans spent nearly $14 billion on alternative therapies. In addition, sales from the natural products industry exceeded $9 billion in 1995 and are increasing every year. Changes that are occurring in the health care field, from increased insurance coverage of alternative therapies to possibly moving away from reductionism in scientific medical research, are all responding to the driving force of the economic marketplace of health care.

If we extend the analogy of Detroit—incorporating new viable ideas and building a better car as a result of losing market share—then health care will improve by adding alternative therapies to the available medical choices. Cost savings to managed care companies for including alternative therapies can be the engine driving alternative therapies into complementary medicine.

CONCLUSION

Alternative medicine is not a passing fad. It is a growing economic player in the health care marketplace, responding to massive consumer demand. It is gaining official legitimation in the political arena and is attracting the attention of biomedical practitioners, who are themselves seeking training in alternative techniques and practices. Although the pace of change is slow, it is occurring. Larry Dossey noted:

> Thirty years ago, people who were interested in diet and exercise were called health nuts. Today, doctors act as if they had invented diet and exercise. Thirty years from now we may see the same kind of change regarding a variety of alternative therapies. (cited in Callahan, 1995, p. 90)

Although change is threatening and often resisted, an increasing number of physicians and nurses and other biomedical practitioners are using and/or becoming familiar with the positive aspects of some alternative therapies. A leveling among professions through the use of similar techniques is occurring. Cooperation among practitioners might gradually increase cooperation between biomedical and alternative practitioners. This approach offers the best solution for providing affordable preventive health and medical care to an increasingly aging population. Continuation and integration of this trend could prove synergistic.

Synergism in science does appear productive to help solve health problems that remain elusive. For example, the "war on cancer," which began in the early 1970s was supported by private citizens and American political leaders who assumed that the "war" could be won in a few years, given sufficient funds to conduct research. Some extraordinary insights have emerged, but many patients with cancer still cannot be cured (Hiatt, 1987, p. 167). Recent advances in treatment of certain types of cancers (e.g., Hodgkin's disease, testicular cancer, and pediatric acute lymphocytic leukemia) have high success rates (M. S. Gordon, radiation oncologist, interview by author, February 1, 1997). Although overall cancer mortality is for the first time following a downward trend in the United States (American Cancer Society, 1997), the high expectations of biomedical science have not been fulfilled. Public disenchantment with science also has been a factor in shrinking governmental support for biomedical research. There is the realization that support does not immediately lead to economic or health benefits. There are gaps in understanding and in treating many ills, pointing to the limits of modern biomedicine.

Analysts contend that biomedical research problems and resource allocation are too restrictive, singular in approach, and limited in answering the pressing health research problems of our country.

> It is a peculiar logic which encourages attempted medical cure of cancer when existing knowledge indicates that the vast majority of human neoplasm (about 80 to 90%) have their genesis in environmental factors such as the food we eat, the water we drink, the air we breathe, self-indulgent habits . . . and even the occupations we choose." (Miller & Stokes, 1987, pp. 346–347).

Negative synergistic reactions from long-term exposure to environmental toxins may account for the increase in breast cancer, yet the scientific community has resisted taking a serious look at the issue (Weil, 1996). Even those who set the standards on toxic levels for pesticide application do not know what safe levels are. Addressing these questions is critical if progress is to be made in finding cures for cancer and other diseases and illnesses. How can this be accomplished?

One way forward is to develop strategies that may have a synergistic effect. These strategies could include (1) interdisciplinary research, (2) clinical and nonclinical studies, (3) research that is both qualitative and quantitative, (4) studies on both groups and individuals, and (5) studies comparing the effects of biomedical and alternative practices for similar conditions. Some of these strategies could be tried within either alternative or biomedical paradigms, but many could borrow from both approaches.

Optimal allocation of scarce health resources would benefit greatly from more interdisciplinary research. It appears that an interdisciplinary approach to basic research, which does not necessarily have to be connected to clinical medicine, is most fruitful. Serendipitous results from basic research in other fields have led to major breakthroughs in medicine. An example is cisplatin, an effective anticancer drug discovered by Barnett Rosenberg, a physicist who was interested in the effects of electrical currents on cell division in bacteria (Hiatt, 1987, p. 167). Another is the development of new anticancer agents by George Pettit, a biochemist who is interested in syntheses of naturally occurring anticancer agents from marine animals, plants, and arthropods (L. Gordon, academic dean, College of Liberal Arts and Sciences, Arizona State University, interview by author, September 10, 1996). These kinds of developments—addressing the important research questions, including those that have been neglected (e.g., environmental and public health factors) and those that have been omitted (e.g., the mind, spirit, and emotions)—provide the most fruitful direction toward solving many human health problems.

In this book it is argued that medicine is undergoing a paradigm expansion, ultimately to form complementary medicine. The change has been initiated by Americans who express dissatisfaction with the limitations of biomedicine with their "feet." They do not wait for scientific validation, which has been blocked from testing both philosophically and financially. Instead, many people seek help and treatment where they can find it. As in any consumer exchange, the buyer must beware. Educating oneself and taking responsibility for one's own health will bring the best results in alternative therapies and in biomedicine. A cooperative, team approach to preventing, treating, and curing health problems shows more promise than does exclusivity or the dogma of any one approach. Only with an expanded vision of health and healing will health care reform become a reality.

References

Abbott, A. (1988). *The system of professions.* Chicago: University of Chicago Press.

Abrams, R. (1985). *Send us a lady physician: Women doctors in America, 1935–1920.* New York: Norton.

Achterberg, J. (1988, January/February). A field guide to health care alternatives. *Utne Reader,* pp. 74–75.

Acupuncture insurance? (1996, April 15). *U.S. News and World Report,* p. 82.

Albuquerque, K. (1979). Folk medicine in the South Carolina sea islands. In M. S. Varner (Ed.), *Proceedings of a Symposium on Culture and Health: Implications for health policy in rural South Carolina* (pp. 33–79). Charleston, SC: College of Charleston, Center for Metropolitan Affairs and Public Policy.

Alster, K. B. (1989). *The holistic health movement.* Tuscaloosa: University of Alabama Press.

Alternative medicine: The facts. (1994). *Consumer Reports, 59*(1), 51–59.

Alvarado, A. L. (1978). Utilization of ethnomedical practitioners and concepts within the framework of Western medicine. In *Modern medicine and medical anthropology in the United States–Mexico border population* (Scientific Publication No. 359). Washington DC: Pan American Health Organization.

AM advisory council meets new OAM staff and reviews progress. (1995, December). *Complementary and Alternative Medicine at the NIH, 2*(5–6), 1, 6–7.

American Association of Health Plans. (1996). *State penetration rates.* Washington, DC: American Association of Health Plans.

American Cancer Society. (1997, January/February). Cancer statistics 1997. *CA: Cancer Journal for Americans, 47*(1), 2–4.

American College of Obstetrics and Gynecology. (1975). *Statement of policy.* Chicago: American College of Obstetrics and Gynecology.

American College of Obstetrics and Gynecology. (1979). *Statement of policy.* Chicago: American College of Obstetrics and Gynecology.

American Holistic Medical Association. (1996). *About the AHMA.* Raleigh, NC: American Holistic Medical Association.

American Medical Association. (1966). *House of Delegates statement.* Chicago: American Medical Association.

AMPAC meeting covers range of issues, Jonas marks year at OAM. (1996, July). *Complementary and Alternative Medicine at the NIH, 3*(2), 1, 7.

Anderson, M. (1996, March). Larry Dossey MD is finding common ground between alternative and conventional medicine. *Natural Foods Merchandiser, 17*(3), 48–52.

Armstrong, D., & Armstrong, E. M. (1991). *The great American medicine show.* New York: Prentice Hall.

Arnold, M. (1992, June). 1991 NFM's 11th annual market overview. *Natural Foods Merchandiser, 13*(5), 1.

Ayanian, J. Z., & Epstein, A. M. (1991). Differences in the use of procedures between women and men hospitalized for coronary heart disease. *New England Journal of Medicine, 325,* 221–225.

Baar, K. (1995). Insurance coverage for all healthcare. *Natural Health, 25,* 74, 76, 78.

Bachelor, A. (1991). Comparison and relationship to outcome of diverse dimensions of the helping alliance as seen by client and therapist. *Psychotherapy, 28,* 534–549.

Baer, H. (1992). The potential rejuvenation of American naturopathy as a consequence of the holistic health movement. *Medical Anthropology, 13,* 369–383.

Baer, L. (1994a). *Alternative health care in the 1990s: The influence of legal constraints on the locational behavior of acupuncturists, chiropractors, and homeopaths.* Unpublished master's thesis, Virginia Polytechnic Institute and State University, Blacksburg.

Baer, L. (1994b). An overview of the influence of legal constraints on the locational behavior of alternative health providers. In J. Frazier, B. Epstein, F. Schoolmaster, & K. Jones (Eds.), *Papers and Proceedings of Applied Geography Conferences* (vol. 17, pp. 101–108). Kent, OH: Kent State University.

Bailar, J. C., III, & Smith, E. M. (1986). Progress against cancer? *New England Journal of Medicine, 314,* 1226–1232.

Balshem, M. (1991). Cancer, control and causality: Talking about cancer in a working-class community. *American Ethnologist, 17,* 152–175.

Barker, J. (1996, July 31). Cancer drug sought for ill son. *Arizona Republic,* pp. A1, A9.

Barrett-Lennard, G. T. (1986). The relationship inventory now. In L. S. Greenberg & W. Pinsof (Eds.), *The psychotherapeutic process: A research handbook* (pp. 439–476). New York: Guilford Press.

Basham, A. L. (1976). The practice of medicine in ancient and medieval India. In *Asian medical systems* (pp. 18–43). Berkeley: University of California Press.

Bastian, H. (1993). Personal beliefs and alternative childbirth choices: A survey of 552 women who planned to give birth at home. *Birth, 20,* 186–192.

Beinfield, H., & Korngold, E. (1991). *Between heaven and earth: A guide to Chinese medicine.* New York: Ballantine.

Bellavite, P., & Signorini, A. (1995). *Homeopathy: Frontier in medical science, experimental studies and theoretical foundations.* Berkeley, CA: North Atlantic Press.

Berman, M., Krishna Singh, B., Lao, L., Singh, B. B., Ferentz, K. S., & Hartnoll, S. M. (1995, September/October). Physicians' attitudes toward complementary or alternative medicine: A regional survey. *Alternative Medicine, 8,* 361–366.

Black Elk, W., & Lyon, W. S. (1990). *Black Elk: The sacred ways of a Lakota.* San Francisco: Harper and Row.

Boddy, J. (1989). *Wombs and alien spirits: Women, men, and the Zar cult in northern Sudan.* Madison: University of Wisconsin Press.

Bonham, G. S., & Corder, L. S. (1981). *NMCES household interview instruments: Instruments and procedures* (1). Rockville, MD: U.S. Department of Health and Human Services.

Bordin, E. S. (1979). The generalizability of the psychoanalytic concept of the working alliance. *Psychotherapy: Theory, Research, and Practice, 126,* 252–260.

Borkan, J., Neher, J. O., Anson, O., & Smoker, B. (1994). Referrals for alternative therapies. *Journal of Family Practice, 39,* 545–550.

Borré, K. (1990–93). *Field notes from project on physicians using complementary medicines* (unpublished). Harrisburg, PA.

Bracht, V. (1931). Texas in 1848 (Frank Schmidt, Trans.). San Antonio, TX: Naylor Co. (Original work published 1849.)

Bradley, R. (1974). *Husband-coached childbirth.* New York: Harper and Row.

Brennan, B. A. (1988). *Hands of light: A guide to healing through the human energy field.* New York: Bantam Books.

Brown, C. (1995, July 30). The experiments of Dr. Oz. *New York Times Magazine,* pp. 21–23.

Brown, H., Cassileth, B. R., Lewis, J. P., & Renner, J. H. (1994, June 15). Alternative medicine—or quackery? *Patient Care,* pp. 83–98.

Brown, L. A. (1968). *Diffusion processes and location* (Bibliography Series No. 4). Philadelphia: Regional Science Research Institute.

Budd, S., & Sharma, U. (Eds.). (1994). *The healing bond: The patient-practitioner relationship and therapeutic responsibility.* London: Routledge.

Burrow, J. (1963). *A.M.A.: Voice of American medicine*. Baltimore: Johns Hopkins University Press.

Burton Goldberg Group. (1995). *Alternative medicine: The definitive guide*. Fife, WA: Future Medicine Publishing.

Cairns, J. (1985). The treatment of diseases and the war against cancer. *Scientific American, 253*(5), 51–59.

Callahan, J. (1995, January/February). Studying the alternatives. *New Age Journal*, pp. 83–90.

Campion, E. W. (1993, January 28). Why unconventional medicine? *New England Journal of Medicine, 328*, 282–283.

Cannon, W. B. (1942). *The wisdom of the body*. New York: Norton.

Caplan, R. L. (1988). Holistic healers in the United States and the changing health care environment. *Holistic Medicine, 3*, 167–174.

Caplan, R. L., & Scarpaci, J. (1989). The consequences of increased competition on alternative health care practitioners in the United States. *Holistic Health, 4*, 325–335.

Cassedy, J. H. (1991). *Medicine in America: A short history*. Baltimore: Johns Hopkins University Press.

Cassidy, C. M. (1994). Unraveling the ball of string: Reality, paradigms, and the study of alternative medicine. *Advances: Journal of Mind-Body Health, 10*, 5–31.

Chabon, I. (1966). *Awake and aware: Participating in childbirth through psychoprophylaxis*. New York: Delacorte Press.

Chin, S. Y. (1992). This, that, and the other: Managing illness in a first-generation Korean family. *Western Journal of Medicine, 157*, 305–309.

Chowka, P. B. (1994, May). *National health care reform and alternative medicine: Never the twain shall meet*. Los Angeles: Whole Life Times.

Christensen, J. (1981). The uncertain application of the right of privacy in personal medical decisions: The laetrile cases. *Ohio State Law Journal, 42*, 523.

Chu, C. M. (1993). *Reproductive health beliefs and practices of Chinese and Australian women*. Taipei: National Taiwan University, Women's Research Program, Population Studies Centre.

Clark, J. (1993). Alternative medicine is catching on. *Kiplinger's Personal Finance Magazine, 47*(1), 98–99.

Clouser, K. D., & Hufford, D. J. (1993). Nonorthodox healing systems and their knowledge claims. *Journal of Medicine and Philosophy, 18*, 101–106.

Coady, N. F. (1991). The association between complex types of therapist interventions and outcomes in psychodynamic psychotherapy. *Research on Social Work Practice 1*(3), 257–277.

Cohen, S. B., & Kalsbeek, W. D. (1981). *NMCES estimation and sampling variances in the household survey: Instruments and procedures* (2). Rockville, MD: U.S. Department of Health and Human Services.

Colgate, M. A. (1995, Spring). Gaining insurance coverage for alternative therapies. *Journal of Health Care Marketing, 15*(1), 24–28.

Committee on Assessing Alternative Birth Settings. (1983). *Research issues in the assessment of birth settings.* Washington, DC: National Academy Press.

Complementary Care Center. (1996). *Operating documents.* New York: Columbia University.

Complementary, not alternative. (1996, February). *Reporter, 7*(1), 6.

Congressional Quarterly. (1992). Alternative medicine: Unproven treatments gain followers, draw warnings of quackery. *CQ Researcher, 2*(4), 73–96.

Cooper, R. A., & Stoflet, S. J. (1996). Trends in the education and practice of alternative medicine clinicians. *Health Affairs, 15*(3), 226–238.

Corry, J. M. (1983). *Consumer health: Facts, skills and decisions.* Belmont, CA: Wadsworth.

Coulter, H. L. (1975, 1977, 1981). *Divided legacy: A history of schism in medical thought* (vols 1–3). Berkeley, CA: North Atlantic Press.

Coulter, H. L. (1982). *Divided legacy: The conflict between homeopathy and the American Medical Association.* Richmond, CA: North Atlantic Books.

Cowley, G., King, P., Hager, M., & Rosenberg, D. (1995). Going mainstream. *Newsweek, 125,* 56–57.

Crellin, J. K. (1987). Folklore and medicines—medical interfaces: A kaleidoscope and challenge. In J. Scarborough (Ed.), *Folklore and folk medicines* (pp. 110–121). Madison, WI: American Institute of the History of Pharmacy.

Curtin, L. S. M. (1947). *Healing herbs of the Upper Rio Grande.* Santa Fe, NM: Laboratory of Anthropology.

Davis-Floyd, R. E. (1992). *Birth as an American rite of passage.* Berkeley: University of California Press.

Davis-Floyd, R. E., & Davis, E. (1996, June). Intuition as authoritative knowledge in midwifery and home birth. *Medical Anthropology Quarterly, 10*(2), 237–269.

De Witt, P. M. (1993). The birth business. *American Demographics, 15,* 44–49.

Declercq, E. R. (1992). The transformation of American midwifery: 1975 to 1988. *American Journal of Public Health, 82,* 680–684.

DeVries, R. G. (1985). *Regulating birth.* Philadelphia: Temple University Press.

Dick-Reed, G. (1959). *Childbirth without fear: The principles and practices of natural childbirth.* New York: Harper and Row.

Dossey, B. M., Keegan, L., Guzzetta, C. E., & Kolkmeier, L. G. (1995). *Holistic nursing: A handbook for practice* (2nd ed). Gaithersburg, MD: Aspen Publishers.

Dossey, L. (1984). *Beyond illness: Discovering the experience of health.* Boulder, CO: New Science Library/Shambhala.

Drury, N. (1983). *Healers, quacks or mystics: A personal exploration of alternative medicine.* Sydney: Hale and Iremonger.

Duke, J. A. (1986). *Handbook of northeastern medicinal plants.* Lincoln, MA: Quarterman Press.

Dunn, F. L. (1976). Traditional Asian medicine and cosmopolitan medicine as adaptive systems. In *Asian medical systems: A comparative study* (pp. 133–158). Berkeley: University of California Press.

Durand, A. M. (1992). The safety of home birth: The farm study. *American Journal of Public Health, 82,* 450–452.

Dyck, I. (1995). Putting chronic illness "in place": Women immigrants' accounts of their health care. *Geoforum, 26,* 247–260.

Editors of the University of California–Berkeley Wellness Letter. (1995). *New wellness encyclopedia.* Berkeley, CA: Houghton Mifflin.

Edwards, M. (1988). Dynamic psychotherapy when both patient and therapist are black. In A. Coner-Edwards & J. Spurlick (Eds.), *Black families in crisis: The middle class* (pp. 61–75). New York: Brunner/Mazel.

Egan, T. (1996, January 3). Seattle area giving natural medicine a chance to come in from the fringe. *New York Times,* p. A10.

Ehrenreich, B., & English, D. (1973). *Witches, nurses and midwives: A history of women healers.* Old Westbury, NY: Feminist Press.

Eisenberg, D. M., Kessler, R. C., Foster, C., Norlock, F. E., Calkins, D. R., & Delbanco, T. L. (1993). Unconventional medicine in the United States: Prevalence, costs and patterns of use. *New England Journal of Medicine, 328,* 246–252.

Emerich, M. (1996, June). Industry growth: 22.6%. *Natural Foods Merchandiser, 17*(6), 1, 22.

Engebretson, J. (1996, Summer). Comparison of nurses and alternative healers. *Image, 28*(2), 95–99.

Evers, M. (1988). *Unconventional cancer treatments.* Washington, DC: Office of Technology Assessment.

Fairfoot, P. (1987). Alternative therapies: The BMA knows best? *Journal of Social Policy, 16,* 383–390.

Federal Trade Commission v. Pharmtech Research, Inc., 576 F. Supp. 294 (D.D.C., 1983).

Federation of Chiropractic Licensing Boards. (1993). *Official directory: Chiropractic licensure and practice statistics, 1993–1994 issue.* Greeley, CO: Federation of Chiropractic Licensing Boards.

Federation of Chiropractic Licensing Boards. (1995). *Official directory: Chiropractic licensure and practice statistics, 1995–1996 issue.* Greeley, CO: Federation of Chiropractic Licensing Boards.

Ferguson, T. (1996). *Health online.* Reading, MA: Addison-Wesley.

Fishman, B. M., Bobo, M., Kosub, K., & Womeodu, R. J. (1993). Cultural issues in serving minority populations: Emphasis on Mexican Americans and African Americans. *American Journal of Medical Sciences, 306*(3), 160–166.

Flexner, A. (1910). *Medical education in the United States and Canada* (Bulletin No. 4). New York: Carnegie Endowment for the Advancement of Teaching.

Fost, D. (1990). Nevada without gambling. *American Demographics, 12,* 47–49.

Foulks, E. F., & Pena, J. M. (1995). Ethnicity and psychotherapy: A component in the treatment of cocaine addiction in African Americans. *Cultural Psychiatry, 18*(3), 607–620.

Fox, K. (1995). Anthropology's hoodoo museum. *Culture, Medicine and Psychiatry, 19,* 409–421.

Frankfort, E. (1972). *Vaginal politics.* New York: Quadrangle Books.

Fugh-Berman, A. (1993). The case for "natural" medicine. *Nation, 257*(7), 240–244.

Fulder, S. (1986). A new interest in complementary (alternative) medicine: Towards pluralism in medicine? *Impact of Science on Society, 143,* 235–243.

Gail, M. H. (1996). Statistics in epidemiology. *Journal of the American Statistical Association, 91*(433), 1–13.

Gallup, G. H., & Bezilla, R. (1996, July 7). Midwest middle-of-road on religion. *New York Times* special features, reprinted in the *Arizona Republic,* p. F15.

Gardner, M. (1957). *Fads and fallacies in the name of science* (2nd ed.). New York: Dover Publications.

Garloch, K. (1993, December 18). N.C. opens to alternative medicine: Law changes status of unusual remedies. *Charlotte Observer,* p. 1C.

Geiser, S. W. (1945). *Horticulture and horticulturalists in early Texas.* Dallas, TX: Southern Methodist University Press.

General information package. (1995, June). Office of Alternative Medicine, National Institutes of Health. Rockville, MD: OAM.

Gesler, W. M. (1988). The place of chiropractors in health care delivery: A case study of North Carolina. *Social Science and Medicine, 26,* 785–792.

Gesler, W. M. (1991). *The cultural geography of health care.* Pittsburgh: University of Pittsburgh Press.

Gevitz, N. (Ed.). (1988). *Other healers: Unorthodox medicine in America.* Baltimore: Johns Hopkins University Press.

Gillett, G. (1994). Beyond the allopathic: Heresy in medicine and social science. *Social Science and Medicine, 39,* 1125–1131.

Gilman, S. C., Justice, J., Saepharn, K., & Charles, G. (1992). Use of traditional and modern health services by Laotian refugees. *Western Journal of Medicine, 157*(3), 310–315.

Glymour, C., & Stalker, D. (1983). Engineers, cranks, physicians, magicians. *New England Journal of Medicine, 308,* 960–964.

Gold, J., & Anastasi, J. (1995). Education opportunities in alternative/complementary medicine for nurses. *Journal of Alternative and Complementary Medicine, 1,* 399–401.

Goldstein, M. S., Sutherland, C. E., Jaffe, D. T., & Wilson, J. (1987). Holistic physicians: Implications for the study of the medical profession. *Journal of Health and Social Behavior, 28,* 103–119.

Goldstein, M. S., Sutherland, C. E., Jaffe, D. T., & Wilson, J. (1988). Holistic physicians and family practitioners: Similarities, differences and implications for health policy. *Social Science and Medicine, 26,* 853–861.

Gomez, G. E., & Gomez, E. A. (1985). Folk healing among Hispanic Americans. *Public Health Nursing, 2*(4), 245–249.

Gonzales, M. L., & Emmons, D. W. (Eds.). (1988). *Socioeconomic characteristics of medical practice.* Chicago: American Medical Association, Center for Health Policy Research.

Gonzalez-Swafford, M. J., & Gutierrez, M. G. (1983). Ethnomedical beliefs and practices of Mexican Americans. *Nurse Practitioner, 8,* 29–34.

Good, C. M. (1977). Traditional medicine: An agenda for medical geography. *Social Science and Medicine, 11,* 705–713.

Goodwin, J. (1997). A health insurance revolution. *New Age Journal's Guide to Holistic Health 1997–1998, Special Edition,* pp. 66–69.

Gordon, J. S. (1980). The paradigm of holistic medicine. In A. C. Hustings, J. Fadiman, & J. S. Gordon (Eds.), *Health for the whole person.* Boulder, CO: Westview Press.

Gordon, R. J. (1990). The effects of malpractice insurance on certified nurse-midwives. *Journal of Nurse-Midwifery, 35*(2), 99–106.

Gordon, R. J., & Nienstedt, B. C. (1992, October). *Alternative health care: An expanding piece of the economic pie.* Paper presented at the meeting of the 15th Annual Applied Geography Conference, Denton, TX.

Gould-Martin, K., & Ngin, C. (1981). Chinese Americans. In A. Harwood (Ed), *Ethnicity and medical care.* Cambridge, MA: Harvard University Press.

Griffin, K. (1995, October). Alternative care: Finally some coverage. *Health,* p. 106.

Groesbeck, C. J. (1975). The archetypal image of the wounded healer. *Journal of Analytic Psychology, 20*(2), 122–145.

Guthrie, A. F. (1991). Intuiting the process of another: Symbolic, rational transformations of experience. *International Journal of Personal Construct Psychology, 4,* 273–279.

Hagerstrand, T. (1968). *Innovation diffusion as a spatial process.* Chicago: University of Chicago Press.

Hall, J. A., Epstein, A. M., DeCiantis, M. L., & McNeil, B. J. (1993). Physicians' liking for their patients: More evidence for the role of affect in medical care. *Health Psychology, 12*(2), 140–146.

Hall, J. A., Roter, D. L., & Katz, N. R. (1988). Meta-analysis of correlates of provider behavior in medical encounters. *Medical Care, 26*, 657–675.

Hamel, R., & Schreiner, T. (1990). Equity refugees. *American Demographics, 12*, 58.

Hamlyn, E. (1979). *The healing art of homeopathy: The organon of Samuel Hahnemann.* New Canaan, CT: Keats Publishing.

Hancock, L. (1994). *Internet/Bitnet Health Sciences Resources.* Retrieved from the Internet/Alternative medicine.

Hansen, P. A. (1991). A suggested medical curriculum for learning about complementary medicine. *Journal of the Royal Society of Medicine, 84*, 702–703.

Harkin, T. (1995, March). The third approach. *Alternative Therapies, 1*(1), 71.

Harner, E. J., & Slater, P. B. (1980). Identifying medical regions using hierarchical clustering. *Social Science and Medicine, 14D*, 3–10.

Harwood, A. (1977). *Rx: Spiritist as needed.* New York: Wiley.

Hassenger, E. W. (1992). *Rural health organization: Social networks and regionalization.* Ames: Iowa State University Press.

Hassinger, E. W., & Hastings, D. V. (1975). Changes in number and location of health practitioners in a 20-county rural area of Missouri. *Public Health Reports, 90*, 313–318.

Hayes-Bautista, D. E. (1978). Chicano patients and medical practitioners: A sociology of knowledge paradigm of lay-professional interaction. *Social Science and Medicine, 12*, 83-90.

Heins, H. C., Nance, N. W., McCarthy, B. J., & Efird, C. M. (1990). A randomized trial of nurse-midwifery prenatal care to reduce low birth weight. *Obstetrics and Gynecology, 75*, 341–345.

Helping people manage pain. (1996). *In Research and scholarship at the University of Virginia School of Nursing* (p. 10). Charlottesville: University of Virginia.

Henry, W. P., Schact, T. E., & Strupp, H. H. (1986). Structural analysis of social behavior: Application to a study of interpersonal processes in differential psychotherapeutic outcome. *Journal of Consulting and Clinical Psychology, 54*, 27–31.

Hiatt, H. H. (1987). *America's health in the balance: Choice or chance?* New York: Harper and Row.

Higginbotham, J. C., Trevino, F. M., & Ray, L. (1990). Utilization of curanderos by Mexican Americans—Prevalence and predictors, Findings from the HHANES 1982–84. *American Journal of Public Health, 80*(Suppl.), 32–35.

Hinton, V. (1983). Foreword. In Neville Drury, *Healers, quacks or mystics: A personal exploration of alternative medicine* (pp. 8–11). Sydney: Hale and Iremonger.

Horvath, A. D., & Greenberg, L. S. (1986). The development of the working alliance inventory. In L. Greenberg & W. Pinsof (Eds.), *The psychotherapeutic process: A research handbook* (pp. 529–556). New York: Guilford Press.

Hudson, C. (1979). *Black drink, A Native American tea.* Athens: University of Georgia Press.

Hulke, M. (1979). Foreword. In M. Hulke (Ed.), *Encyclopedia of alternative medicine and self-help* (pp. 11–12). New York: Schocken Books.

Hulkrantz, A. (1985). The shaman and the medicine man. *Social Science and Medicine, 20,* 511–515.

In re George A. Guess, MD (1990), Supreme Court of North Carolina, 393 S. E. 2d 833.

Inglis, B., & West, R. (1983). *The alternative health guide.* New York: Knopf.

Injunctive Order against AMA (1987). *Journal of the American Medical Association, 259,* 1.

Ivey, A. E. (1987). The multicultural practice of therapy: Ethics, empathy, and dialectics. *Journal of Social and Clinical Psychology, 5*(2), 195–204.

Jacobs, J. J. (1995, January). Building bridges between two worlds: NIH's Office of Alternative Medicine. *Academic Medicine, 70*(1), 40–41.

Janiger, O., & Goldberg, P. (1994). *A different kind of healing: Why mainstream doctors are embracing alternative medicine.* New York: Putnam.

Jantsch, E. (1980). *The self-organizing universe.* New York: Pergamon.

Jenkins, S. (1993, June 26). Turn back to the quacks (p. 14). *The Times* (London).

Johnson, I. (1982). Introduction: The history of the 1906 pure food and drug act and the meat inspection act. *Food, Drug and Cosmetic Law Journal, 37,* 310–312.

Jones, J. (1995, August 20). Quacks no more as therapists get NHS approval (p. 8). *The Observer* (London).

Jordan, T. G. (1966). *German seed in Texas soil.* Austin: University of Texas Press.

Kao, F. F., & McRae, G. (1986). Chinese medicine in America: The rocky road to ecumenical medicine. *Impact of Science on Society, 143,* 263–273.

Kaufman, M. (1971). *Homeopathy in America: The rise and fall of a medical heresy.* Baltimore: Johns Hopkins University Press.

Kay, M. A. (1977). Health and illness in a Mexican-American barrio. In *Ethnic medicine in the Southwest* (pp. 99–166). Tucson: University of Arizona Press.

Kearney, H., & Rosch, P. J. (1985). Holistic medicine and technology: A modern dialectic. *Social Science and Medicine, 21,* 1405–1409.

Kelly, T. A., & Strupp, H. H. (1992). Patient and therapist values in psychotherapy: Perceived changes, assimilation, similarity, and outcome. *Journal of Consulting and Clinical Psychology, 60,* 34–40.

Kerr, H. D. (1993). White liver: A cultural disorder resembling AIDS. *Social Science and Medicine, 36,* 609–614.

Kiesler, D. J., & Watkins, L. M. (1989). Interpersonal complementarity and the therapeutic alliance: A study of relationship in psychotherapy. *Psychotherapy, 26,* 183–194.

Kimber, C. (1972). *Field notes in the Lower Rio Grande Valley of Texas.* Unpublished manuscript.

Kimber, C. (1973). Native and exotic plants in the folk medicine of the Texas borderlands. *Proceedings of the Association of American Geographers, 5,* 130–133.

Kimber, C. (1985). *Field notes in West Indian islands.* Unpublished manuscript.

King, D. E., & Bushwick, B. (1994). Beliefs and attitudes of hospital inpatients about faith healing and prayer. *Journal of Family Practice, 39,* 349–352.

King, I. M. (1967). *John O. Meuseback: German colonizer in Texas.* Austin: University of Texas Press.

King, L. J. (1984). *Central place theory* (Scientific Geography Series, Vol. 1). Beverly Hills: Sage Publications.

Klatz, R. & Kahn, C. (1997). *Parade Magazine,* April 20, 20–23.

Kleinman, A. (1980). *Patients and healers in the context of culture: An exploration of the borderland between anthropology, medicine, and psychiatry.* Berkeley: University of California Press.

Kloss, J. (1939). *Back to Eden.* Loma Linda, CA: Back to Eden Books.

Knipschild, P., Kleijnen, J., & Ter Riet, G. (1990). Belief in the efficacy of alternative medicine among general practitioners in the Netherlands. *Social Science and Medicine, 31,* 625–626.

Kohler, D. L., Bellenger, D. N., & Whyte, G. E. (1990). The role of birthing centers in hospital marketing. *Health Care Management Review, 15,* 71–77.

Kohut, H. (1984). *How does analysis cure?* (A. Goldberg, Ed., with the collaboration of P. E. Stepansky). Chicago: University of Chicago Press.

Kolata, G. (1996a, June 17). Alternative medicine: Beyond the mainstream. *The New York Times,* pp. A1, C11.

Kolata, G. (1996b, June 18). Alternative medicine: Research without results. *The New York Times,* pp. A1, B7.

Koss-Chioino, J. D. (1992). *Women as healers, women as patients.* Boulder, CO: Westview.

Koss-Chioino, J. D. (1995). Traditional and folk approaches among ethnic minorities. In J. F. Aponte, R. R. Rivers, & J. Wohl (Eds.), *Psychological intervention and treatment of ethnic minorities: Concepts, issues, and methods,* pp. 145–163. Needham Heights, MA: Allyn and Bacon.

Koss-Chioino, J. D. (1996). The experience of spirits: Ritual healing as transactions of emotion (Puerto Rico). In W. Andritzky (Ed.), *Yearbook of cross-cultural medicine and psychotherapy, Vol. 1993, Ethnopsychotherapy* pp. 251–271. Berlin: Verlag fur Wissemschaft und Bildung.

Koss-Chioino, J. D., & Vargas, L. A. (1992). Through the cultural looking glass: A model for understanding culturally responsive psychotherapies. In L. A. Vargas & J. D. Koss-Chioino (Eds.), *Working with culture: Psychotherapeutic interventions with ethnic minority children and adolescents* (pp. 1–22). San Francisco: Jossey-Bass.

Kramer B. J. (1992). Health and aging of urban Native American Indians. *Western Journal of Medicine, 157*(3), 281–285.

Krieger, D. (1979). *The therapeutic touch: How to use your hands to help or to heal.* Englewood Cliffs, NJ: Prentice-Hall.

Krieger, D. (1981). *Foundations for holistic health nursing practices: The renaissance nurse.* Philadelphia: Lippincott.

Kuhn, T. S. (1970). *The structure of scientific revolutions* (2nd ed.). Chicago: University of Chicago Press.

Kviz, F. J. (1984). Bias in a directory sample for a mail survey of rural households. *Public Opinion Quarterly, 48,* 801–806.

Laguerre, M. (1987). *Afro-Caribbean folk medicine.* South Hadley, MA: Bergin and Garvey.

Langs, R. (1978). *Technique in transition.* New York: Jason Aronson.

Lannie, D. D. (1982). *Folk traditions in medical care of a German Texas community: Gillespie County, Texas.* Unpublished doctoral dissertation, Texas A&M University, College Station.

Last, M. (1990). Professionalization of indigenous healers (pp. 374–395). In T. Johnson & C. Sargent (Eds.), *Medical anthropology: Contemporary theory and method.* New York: Praeger.

Lazarus, E. S. (1988). Theoretical considerations for the study of the doctor-patient relationship: Implications of a perinatal study. *Medical Anthropology Quarterly, 2*(1), 34–58.

Lazlo, J. (1987). *Understanding cancer.* New York: Harper and Row.

Leap of faith in cardiac care. (1995, Fall). *Biomedical Frontiers, 3*(1), 1, 9.

Lehmann, H. (1927). *Nine years among the Indians, 1870–1879.* Austin, TX: Von-Boechmann-Jones.

LeShan, L. (1974). *The medium, the mystic, and the physicist.* New York: Viking.

Lisa, P. J. (1994). *The assault on medical freedom.* Norfolk, VA: Hampton Roads Publishing.

Litoff, J. B. (1978). *American midwives, 1860 to the present.* Westport, CT: Greenwood Press.

Litoff, J. B. (1986). *The American midwife debate: A sourcebook on its modern origins.* New York: Greenwood Press.

Lloyd, C., & Maas, F. (1991). The therapeutic relationship. *British Journal of Occupational Therapy, 54*(3), 111–113.

Lockie, A. (1989). *The family guide to homeopathy.* New York: Simon and Schuster.

Lockie, A., & Geddes, N. (1995). *Homeopathy: The principles, practice and treatment.* London: Dorling Kindersley.

Luborsky, L., McLellan, A. T., Woody, G. E., O'Brien, C. P., & Auerbach, A. (1985). Therapist success and its determinants. *Archives of General Psychiatry, 42,* 602–611.

Lucas, V. A. (1993, June). Birth: Nursing's role in today's choices. *RN,* pp. 38–44.

Lupton, D., Donaldson, C., & Lloyd, P. (1991). Caveat emptor or blissful ignorance? Patients and the consumerist ethos. *Social Science and Medicine, 33,* 559–568.

Lynes, B. (1992). *The healing of cancer.* Wilmington, MA: Marcus Books.

Maduro, R. (1983). Curanderismo and Latino views on disease and curing. *Western Journal of Medicine, 139,* 868–874.

Makulowich, J. S. (1994, July). *Internet Resources on Alternative Medicine.* Retrieved from Internet/Alternative Medicine.

Managed Care Digest. (1995). Kansas City, MO: Marion Merrell Dow.

Mantz, D. (1913). *Mantz papers.* Victoria, TX: Victoria Advocate.

Marsh, W. M., & Hentges, K. (1988). Mexican folk remedies and conventional medical care. *American Family Physician, 37*(3), 257–262.

Marshall, C. L., Hassanein, H. M., Hassanein, R. J., & Marshall, C. L. (1971). Principal components analysis of the distribution of physicians, dentists, and osteopaths in a midwestern state. *American Journal of Public Health, 61,* 1556–1564.

Marziali. E., & Alexander, L. (1991). The power of the therapeutic relationship. *American Journal of Orthopsychiatry, 61,* 383–391.

Mattingly, P. F. (1991). The changing location of physician offices in Bloomington–Normal, Illinois: 1870–1988. *Professional Geographer, 43,* 465–474.

McClenon, J. (1993). The experiential foundations of shamanic healing. *Journal of Medicine and Philosophy, 18,* 107–127.

McDaniels, A. (1991). Differences in training backgrounds of physician acupuncturists and licensed acupuncturists. *AAMA Review, 3*(1), 15–19.

McGaa, E. (Eagle Man). (1990). *Mother Earth spirituality: Native American paths to healing ourselves and our world.* San Francisco: Harper and Row.

McGuire, M. B. (1988). *Ritual healing in suburban America.* New Brunswick, NJ: Rutgers University Press.

McKee, N. (1992). Lexical and semantic pitfalls in the use of survey interviews: An example from the Texas-Mexico border. *Hispanic Journal of Behavioral Sciences, 14,* 353–362.

McKeown, L. A. (1993, April). The healing profession on an alternative mission. *Medical World News,* pp. 48, 49, 53, 54, 60.

McLaughlin, C. (1995, October 9). Alternative therapies: Gaining acceptance in mainstream medicine. *Advance for Physical Therapists*, pp. 10–11, 62.

McRae, G. (1982). A critical overview of U.S. acupuncture regulation. *Journal of Health, Politics, Policy and Law 7*(1), 163–196.

Meade, M. S., Florin, J. W., & Gesler, W. M. (1988). Accessibility and utilization. In M. S. Meade, J. W. Florin, & W. M. Gesler (Eds.), *Medical geography* (pp. 312–313). New York: Guilford Press.

Mechanic, D. (1979). *Future issues in health care.* New York: Free Press.

Media: Natural medicine over the airwaves. (1996, May). *Delicious!*, p. 14.

Medical education and state boards of registration. (1909). *Journal of the American Medical Association, 52*, 1691–1713.

Mehl, L. (1977). Outcomes of 1146 elective home deliveries. *Journal of Reproductive Medicine, 19*, 281–290.

Merchant, R. K. (1996). *Perception of availability of health care by the underserved.* Paper presented at the Annual Conference for the Behavioral Sciences and Medical Education. October 15, 1995, Naples, Florida.

Micozzi, M. S. (Ed.). (1996). *Fundamentals of complementary and alternative medicine.* New York: Churchill Livingstone.

Miller, M. K., & Stokes, C. S. (1987). The medical care system and the protection of health. In M. R. Greenberg (Ed.), *Public health and the environment: The United States experience* (pp. 331–350). New York: Guilford Press.

Mitchell, B. (1995). *Acupuncture and oriental medicine laws.* Washington, DC: National Acupuncture Foundation.

Mitchell, S. (1993). Healing without doctors. *American Demographics, 15*, 46–49.

Mo, B. (1992). Modesty, sexuality, and breast health in Chinese American women. *Western Journal of Medicine, 157*(3), 260–264.

Monmonier, M. (1971). Comparative geography of medical and osteopathic physicians in the United States, 1967. *Pennsylvania Academy of Science, 45*, 121–129.

Monson, N. (1995, May). Alternative medicine education at medical schools: Are they catching on? *Alternative and Complementary Therapies*, pp. 168–170.

Moore, J. S. (1990). Chiropractic in America: The flourishing of a medical pariah. Unpublished doctoral dissertation, University of Virginia, Charlottesville.

Moore, N. (1995, May). Arizona center for health and medicine: A model of integrated healthcare. *Alternative Therapies in Health and Medicine, 1*(2), 17.

Morgan, R. W. (1973). Migration as a factor in the acceptance of medical care. *Social Science and Medicine, 5*, 137–194.

Morrisey, M. A., Sloan, F. A., & Valvona, J. (1988). Defining geographic markets for hospital care. *Law and Contemporary Problems, 51*, 165–194.

Moskowitz, R. (1993, Winter). Why I became a homeopath. *Holistic Medicine*, pp. 22, 23, 27.

Moyers, B. (1995). *Healing and the mind.* New York: Doubleday.

Murray, R. H., & Rubel, A. J. (1992). Physicians and healers: Unwilling partners in health care. *New England Journal of Medicine, 326,* 61–64.

National Center for Homeopathy. (1993). *Directory: Practitioners, study groups, pharmacies and resources.* Alexandria, VA: National Center for Homeopathy.

National Center for Homeopathy. (1996). *Directory: Practitioners, study groups, pharmacies and resources.* Alexandria, VA: National Center for Homeopathy.

National Commission for the Certification of Acupuncture (NCCA). (1993). *1993 Directory of National Board Certified Acupuncturists.* Washington, DC: Author.

National Institutes of Health. (1994). *Alternative medicine: Expanding medical horizons. A report to the National Institutes of Health on alternative medicine systems and practices in the United States* (NIH Publication No. 94-066). Chantilly, Virginia: The Workshop on Alternative Medicine September 14–16, 1992.

National Institutes of Health. (1997). From Internet. gopher:/gopher.nih.gov/11/res/brownbook/resgr.

Newman, M. A. (1994). *Health as expanding consciousness* (2nd ed.). New York: National League for Nursing Press.

Nightingale, F. (1992). *Notes on nursing.* Philadelphia: Lippincott. (Original work published 1859, London: Harrison & Sons.)

NIH panel endorses alternative therapies for chronic pain and insomnia. (1995, December). *Complementary and Alternative Medicine at the NIH, 2*(5–6), 3, 8.

OAM funds eight research centers to evaluate alternative treatments. (1995, December). *Complementary and Alternative Medicine at the NIH, 2*(5–6), 2, 8.

O'Connor, B. B. (1993). The home birth movement in the United States. *Journal of Medicine and Philosophy, 18,* 147–174.

Office of Science Policy and Legislation. Meeting-Unconventional Medical Practices. (1992, June 2). *Federal Register, 57,* 23242.

Orlinsky, D., & Howard, K. (1975). *Varieties of psychotherapeutic experience.* New York: Teachers College Press.

Orlinsky, D. E., Grawe, K., & Parks, B. K. (1994). Process and outcome in psychotherapy: Noch einmal. In A. E. Bergin & S. L. Garfield (Eds.), *Handbook of psychotherapy and behavior change* (4th ed., pp. 270–376). New York: Wiley.

Osborn, A. R. (1990). *The distribution of orthodox and alternative primary health care practitioners in San Diego County.* Unpublished master's thesis, San Diego State University.

Osborn, A. R. (1997). *Considering the alternatives: The geography of unconventional health care in California, Oregon and Washington.* Unpublished doctoral dissertation, University of Oregon, Eugene.

Pappas, G. (1990). Some implications for the study of the doctor-patient relationship interaction: Power structure and agency in the works of Howard Waitzkin and Arthur Kleinman. *Social Science and Medicine, 30,* 199–204.

Patch, F. B., & Holaday, S. D. (1989). Effects of changes in professional liability insurance on certified nurse-midwives. *Journal of Nurse-Midwifery,* 34(3), 131–136.

Pavek, R. R., & Trachtenberg, A. I. (1995). Current status of alternative health practices in the United States. *Contemporary Internal Medicine, 7*(8), 61–71.

Peltz, J. F. (1993, July 28). Insurer to reimburse cost of nonsurgical heart care. *Los Angeles Times,* p. A1.

Perkin, M. R., Pearcy, R. M., & Fraser, J. S. (1994). A comparison of the attitudes shown by general practitioners, hospital doctors and medical students towards alternative medicine. *Journal of the Royal Society of Medicine, 87,* 523–525.

Perrone, B., Stockel, H. H., & Krueger, V. (1989). *Medicine women, curanderas, and women doctors.* Norman, OK: University of Oklahoma Press.

Pert, C. (1995). The chemical communicators. In B. Moyers (Ed.), *Healing and the mind* (pp. 177–193). New York: Main Street Books, Doubleday.

Pescosolido, B. A. (1986). The migration, medical care preferences and the lay referral system: A network theory of role assimilation. *American Sociological Review, 51,* 523–540.

Peters, L. G. (1981). An experiential study of Nepalese shamanism. *Journal of Transpersonal Psychology, 13*(1), 1–26.

Picozzi, M. (1996, March). A retail buyer's guide to supplements: Understanding what to expect from different sales channels can streamline buying and increase customer services. *Natural Foods Merchandiser, 17*(3), 120.

Porkert, M. (1990). *Theoretical foundations of Chinese medicine.* Boston: MIT Press.

Power, R. (1994). 'Only nature heals': A discussion of therapeutic responsibility from a naturopathic point of view. In S. Budd & U. Sharma (Eds.), *The healing bond: The patient-practitioner relationship and therapeutic responsibility* (pp. 193–213). London: Routledge.

Prigogine, I., & Stengers, I. (1984). *Order out of chaos.* New York: Bantam Books.

Quesada, G. M., & Heller, P. L. (1977). Sociocultural barriers to medical care among Mexican Americans in Texas. *Medical Care, 15*(5), 97–101.

Quinn, J. (1994). Caring for the caregiver. In J. Watson (Ed.), *Applying the art and science of human caring* (pp. 63–71). New York: National League for Nursing Press.

Reid, M. (1991). Sisterhood and professionalization: A case study of the American lay midwife. In *Women as healers: Cross-cultural perspectives* (pp. 219–238). New Brunswick, NJ: Rutgers University Press.

Rich, A. (1977). Theft of childbirth. In C. Dreifus (Ed.), *Seizing our bodies: The politics of women's health.* New York: Vintage Books.

Rogler, L. H., Malgady, R. G., Costantino, G., & Blumenthal, R. (1987). What do culturally sensitive mental health services mean? The case of Hispanics. *American Psychologist, 42,* 565–570.

Rooks, J. P., & Haas, J. E. (Eds.). (1986). *Nurse midwifery in America.* Washington, DC: American College of Nurse-Midwives Foundation.

Rosch, P. J. (1981). Holistic medicine: Health care of the future? In L. K. Y. Ng & D. L. Davis (Eds.), *Strategies for public health: Promoting health and preventing disease* (pp. 59–70). New York: Van Nostrand Reinhold.

Rothman, B. K. (1982). *In labor: Women and power in the birthplace.* New York: Norton.

Rowley, B. D., & Baldwin, D. C., Jr. (1984). Assessing rural community resources for health care: The use of health services catchment area economic marketing studies. *Social Science and Medicine, 18,* 525–529.

Russell, C. (1993). *The master trend: How the baby boom generation is remaking America.* New York: Plenum Press.

Ruzek, S. B. (1978). *The women's health movement: Feminist alternatives to medical control.* New York: Praeger.

Sale, D. (1995). *Overview of legislative developments concerning alternative health care in the United States.* Kalamazoo, MI: Fetzer Institute.

Satin, M. (1988, January/February). National holistic health care. *Utne Reader,* pp. 76–79.

Schloendorff v. Society of New York Hospital, 211 N.Y. 125, 129–30 (1914).

Schmidt, M. (1996). *Healing childhood ear infections.* Berkeley, CA: North Atlantic Press.

Schneider, D. (1986). Planned out-of-hospital births, New Jersey, 1978–1980. *Social Science and Medicine, 23,* 1011–1015.

Schrom Dye, N. (1983). Mary Breckenridge, the Frontier Nursing Service and the introduction of nurse-midwifery in the United States. *Bulletin of the History of Medicine, 57,* 485–507.

Schuyler, C. (1992). Florence Nightingale. In F. Nightingale, *Notes on nursing* (pp. 3–17). Philadelphia: Lippincott.

Shannon, G. W., & Dever, G. E. A. (1974). *Health care delivery: Spatial perspectives.* New York: McGraw-Hill.

Snow, L. (1993). *Walkin' over medicine: Traditional health practices in African American life.* Boulder, CO: Westview Press.

Soja, E. (1985). The spatiality of social life: Towards a transformative rethe-orisation. In D. Gregory & J. Urry (Eds.), *Social relations and spatial structures* (pp. 90–127). London: Macmillan.

Steefel, L. (1996, May 25). Shifting mainstream medicine. *Nursing Spectrum, 8*(7), 4, 7–8.

Stein, R. (1973). *Incest and human love: The betrayal of the soul in psychotherapy.* Baltimore: Penguin Books.

Stewart, D., & Stewart, L. (Eds.). (1979). *Compulsory hospitalization or freedom of choice in childbirth?* (Vol. 3). Marble Hill, MO: National Association of Parents and Professionals for Safe Alternatives in Childbirth.

Stimson, R. J. (1981). The provision and use of general practitioner services in Adelaide, Australia: Application of tools of locational analysis and theories of provider and user spatial behaviour. *Social Science and Medicine, 15D,* 27–44.

Sue, D. W., & Sue, D. (1990). *Counseling the culturally different* (2nd ed.). New York: Wiley.

Sue, S. (1988). Psychotherapeutic services for ethnic minorities. *American Psychologist, 43,* 301–308.

Taylor, D. H., & Ricketts, T. C. (1993). Helping nurse-midwives provide obstetrical care in rural North Carolina. *American Journal of Public Health, 83,* 904–905.

Thaden, J. F. (1951). *Distribution of doctors of medicine and osteopaths in Michigan communities* (Special Bulletin No. 370). East Lansing: Michigan State College, Agricultural Experiment Station, Department of Sociology and Anthropology and Social Research Service.

Tiling, M. (1913). *History of the German element in Texas, from 1820–1850.* Houston: Rein and Sons.

Topper, M. D. (1987). The traditional Navajo medicine man: Therapist, counselor, and community leader. *Journal of Psychoanalytic Anthropology, 10,* 217–250.

Trotter, R. T., II, & Chavira, J. A. (1981). *Curanderismo: Mexican American folk healing.* Athens: University of Georgia.

Ullman, D. (1991). *Discovering homeopathic medicine for the 21st century.* Berkeley, CA: North Atlantic Books.

Ullman, D. (1992). *Homeopathic medicines for children and infants.* Los Angeles: Jeremy Tarcher.

Ullman, D. (1995). *The consumer's guide to homeopathy.* New York: Putnam.

Unconventional claims. (1995, October). *Vegetarian Times,* p. 27.

U.S. Bureau of the Census. (1996a, February). *Current population reports, population projections of the U.S. by age, sex, race, and Hispanic origin: 1995–2050* (Series #P25-1130). Washington, DC: U.S. Government Printing Office.

U.S. Bureau of the Census. (1996b). Resident population by age and state: 1995. In *Statistical abstracts of the U.S.* (116th ed.). Washington, DC: U.S. Government Printing Office.

U.S. Department of Health and Human Services. (1994). *Vital statistics of the United States 1990: Vol. 1. Natality.* Hyattsville, MD: National Center for Health Statistics.

U.S. Department of Health and Human Services, Agency for Health Care Policy and Research. (1995). Elderly Asian Americans seldom seek medical care. *Research Activities, 187,* 10–11.

Wallis, R., & Morley, P. (1976). Introduction. In Roy Wallis & Peter Morley (Eds.), *Marginal medicine* (pp. 9–19). London: Peter Owen.

Wardwell, W. I. (1963). Limited, marginal, and quasi-practitioners. In E. Freeman, S. Levine, & L. G. Reeder (Eds.), *Handbook of medical sociology* (pp. 213–239). Englewood Cliffs, NJ: Prentice-Hall.

Wardwell, W. I. (1988). Chiropractors: Evolution to acceptance. In N. Gevitz (Ed.), *Other healers: Unorthodox medicine in America* (pp. 157–191). Baltimore: Johns Hopkins University Press.

Wardwell, W. I. (1994). Alternative medicine in the United States. *Social Science and Medicine, 38,* 1061–1068.

Watson, J. (1988). *Nursing: Human science and human care: A theory of nursing.* New York: National League for Nursing Press.

Weil, A. (1988). *Health and healing.* Boston: Houghton Mifflin.

Weil, A. (1995). *Spontaneous healing: How to discover and enhance your body's natural ability to maintain and heal itself.* New York: Alfred A. Knopf.

Weil, A. (1996, August 20). *Nutrition: Cornerstone of integrative medicine.* Professional Mini-Conference Series. Tucson: University of Arizona College of Medicine.

Weitz, R., & Sullivan, D. (1985). Licensed lay midwifery and the medical model of childbirth. *Sociology of Health and Illness, 7,* 36–54.

Wertz, R. W., & Wertz, D. C. (1977). *Lying-in: A history of childbirth in America.* New York: Free Press.

Wilk v. American Medical Association, 671 F. Supp. 1465 (7th Cir. 1987).

Wish, H. (1960). Turner and the moving of the frontier. In *The American historian* (pp. 181–208). New York: Oxford University Press.

World Health Organization. (1992). *The integration of environmental health into planning for urban development.* Kuala Lumpur, Malaysia: Author.

World Health Organization. (1993). *WHO global strategy for health and environment.* Geneva: Author.

Wright, J. W. (Ed.). (1990). *Universal almanac.* Kansas City, MO: Andrew and McNeel.

Yesalis, C. E., Wallace, R. B., Fisher, W. P., & Tokheim, R. (1980). Does chiropractic utilization substitute for less available medical services? *American Journal of Public Health, 70,* 415–417.

Young, G., & Drife, J. (1992). Therapeutic dilemma: Home birth is an acceptable option: birth should take place in hospital. *Practitioner, 126,* 672–674.

Zaldivar, A., & Smolowitz, J. (1994). Perceptions of the importance placed on religion and folk medicine by non-Mexican American Hispanic adults with diabetes. *Diabetes Educator, 20,* 303–306.

Zwicky, J. F., Hafner, A. W., Barret, S., & Jarvis, W. T. (1993). *Reader's guide to alternative health methods.* Milwaukee, WI: American Medical Association.

Glossary of Alternative Practices
Barbara Cable Nienstedt

EXTERNAL BODY HEALING

Alexander therapists use proper posture and breathing to achieve natural balance and correct problems such as back pain, arthritis, rheumatism, and gastrointestinal and breathing disorders.

Anthroposophic medicine is based on a model of human individuality that includes nature, the soul, and human spirit. It combines biomedicine with homeopathy and naturopathy and advocates the balance of three interdependent parts of the body-mind process: sense-nerve (central nervous system, brain), rhythmic (pulse, heartbeat), and metabolic-limb (digestive, elimination, metabolism).

Applied kinesiology serves mainly as a diagnostic tool by identifying imbalances in the body's organs and glands through weaknesses in specific muscles. Through stimulation or relaxation of these weak muscles it resolves those health problems.

Aston patterning focuses on body symmetry and alignment. Treatment works on movement reeducation, massage and soft tissue bodywork, fitness training, and environmental design.

Body energy therapies are based on different energy models. These models are often incorporated into other alternative therapies, such as oriental *chi*, or *qi*, energy in acupressure; Western energy flow in polarity therapy; and energy healing in therapeutic touch. Massage therapists often incorporate energy work into their sessions.

Bodywork therapies use massage, deep- and soft-tissue manipulation, and energy balancing to reduce pain and stimulate blood and lymph circulation.

Chiropractic manipulates the spine to adjust subluxations (misalignments). This procedure corrects nervous system disorders, alleviates pain, controls addictions, and prevents disease. Chiropractors often advocate nutritional supplements and vitamin therapy in conjunction with spinal adjustments.

Cranialsacral therapy focuses on the central nervous system and the fluid, membranes, and bones comprising it. The therapist monitors the ebb and flow of the system to diagnose dysfunction in its rhythm. Through gentle manipulation, pressure on the troubled spots relieves stress and restores balance to the brain and spinal cord.

Ear coning therapy was used in ancient times by Egyptian pharaohs, Greek oracles and emperors, Aztecs and Mayans. It disappeared from the healing arena until New Age alternative practitioners rediscovered it. Herbal cones approximately one foot in length are lit and inserted into the ear for clearing sinuses and auditory canals. Stress reduction and relaxation are important concomitants.

Energy medicine diagnoses and treats imbalances in energy flows (known as *chi* or *qi* in oriental medicine) with electromagnetic impulses. Based on the meridian system used in acupuncture, various types of computerized electronic instruments are used for restoring bioenergetic balance, thus preventing disease and working as a treatment for ailments.

Environmental medicine, also known as bioecological medicine, links illness to stress, food, chemicals, and environmental sensitivity. Complete nutritional and environmental histories are taken, along with a physical exam. Special attention is paid to yeast, molds, fungi, parasites, and pollen as well as chemical exposure, dental work, and heredity.

Feldenkrais methods recognize self-image as central to healing. Improper breathing and movement, even of the eyes, can seriously impair body function.

Hellerwork is the practice of deep-tissue bodywork and awareness of the mind/body relationship to restructure the body. It also advocates the proper alignment of the body with the gravitational field of the earth.

Hydrotherapy and *hyperthermia* use water in all its forms, from ice to steam, to restore health and prevent disease and are grounded in ancient practice. Hot water stimulates the immune system by causing white cells to go from blood to tissue, where they detoxify and eliminate waste. Cold water constricts blood vessels, reducing inflammation and toning muscles. Hyperthermia therapy induces fever through hot baths, thereby stimulating the immune system and increasing antibodies and interferon.

Iridology analyzes the iris of the eye for signs of disease in the body; it is primarily a diagnostic tool. Iridologists study the shape, color, and quality of the iris tissue; structural patterns; and flecks of pigmentation. Every gland and organ has its own place on the iris. Iridologists can determine physical, physiological, and nutritional deficiencies; stress conditions; and under- and overactive glands. They work with clients to promote good health.

Lepore technique is a system that uses a refined kinesiology (muscle response testing) to locate a metabolic antagonist causing disease. It determines a nutritional antidote to neutralize the metabolic antagonist and prescribes support nutrients that act as catalysts to facilitate absorption of the antidote.

Light therapy activates the body's chemicals through natural sunlight and certain types of artificial light, thereby correcting the negative effects of lighting normally found in homes and offices. Full-spectrum light, bright light, ultraviolet light, and laser light therapies produce beams that enter the eye and are converted into electric impulses. These beams travel along the optic nerve to the brain and activate neurotransmitters in the hypothalamus gland and endocrine system that regulate most bodily functions and, consequently, a person's health.

Magnetic field therapy is also known as *electromagnetic therapy.* It is the use of magnets and electromagnetic devices to penetrate the body in order to eliminate pain, heal broken bones and infections, and relieve stress. The therapy can also stimulate metabolism and increase the amount of oxygen available to the cells. Magnetic field therapy also counters the effect of electromagnetic pollution in the environment.

Metabolic therapy includes an eclectic combination of diet and supplements, detoxification, immune stimulation, herbal medicine, and enzyme therapy aimed at restoring metabolic balance to ward off disease.

Myotherapy applies manual pressure to "trigger points" (excessively sore muscles) for 5 to 7 seconds to relieve pain. The body is divided into five zones from Zone I, the headache zone, to Zone V, the feet and leg zone; pain can be released through self-pressure.

Neural therapy believes illness begins when the individual's energy flow is disrupted. It treats chronic pain, illness, and trauma by injection of anesthetics into acupuncture points, scars, glands, nerves, or other tissues to correct blockages in the body's electrical network. Once the sick cells regain their normal electrical activity, they eliminate toxic wastes that have built up.

Polarity therapy is based on a person's electromagnetic energy currents. Disturbances or blockages along the energy paths result in illness. Removing the blockage through breathing, massage, diet, exercise, hydrotherapy, and holding pressure points resolves the problem.

Reconstructive therapy involves injection of natural substances to stimulate growth of connective tissue surrounding injured or painful joints, tendons, ligaments, and cartilage. Benefits of this treatment include low side effects, no surgery, stimulation of the body's natural healing mechanisms, and permanent results.

Reflexology teaches that the hands and feet contain reflex areas that correspond to all the organs and glands in the body. A picture of the foot provides a map for the body areas, and pressure applied to certain spots corrects the energy flow by breaking up lactic acid buildup and calcium crystals, producing relief from pain and disease.

Rolfing, also known as *structural integration*, posits that the body's structure affects all physiological and psychological processes. Fascial tissues and covering muscles are manually manipulated and stretched by fingers, knuckles, and elbows.

Rosen methods combine touch, deep breathing, and verbal communication to bring about muscular relaxation. Gentle range-of-motion exercises are set to music for psychological and emotional health as well as physical healing and stimulation of the immune system.

Schuessler tissue salts are 12 different cell salts—all that are necessary for perfect health. By proper biochemical balancing, based on homeopathic remedies, the underlying cause of illness and disease and its symptoms will disappear.

Therapeutic massage benefits many conditions of ill health by triggering reflex actions in the body to stimulate organs. It also breaks up muscular waste deposits and stimulates circulation, working effectively on musculoskeletal problems and pain.

Therapeutic touch, contrary to its name, often does not use physical touch. It combines visualization, aura reading, and working 2 to 6 inches from the patient's body to release any obstructions in the patient's energy field. Occasionally, there may be some laying on of hands in more extreme injury.

Trager method reeducates body movement through gentle rhythmical massage and movement exercises. The movements induce a sense of deep relaxation, and increase flexibility and range of motion.

Zone therapy is the precursor to reflexology, using finger pressure points on the hands and mouth instead of the foot to alleviate symptoms of pain and disease.

INTERNAL BODY HEALING

Antineoplaston therapy reprograms defective cells through certain amino acids (polypeptides) called antineoplastons (meaning anti-new growth). Antineoplastons interact with the DNA and take the place of carcinogens that would otherwise occupy the DNA strand. As this occurs, the antineoplastons redirect the DNA into normal reproduction.

Applied nutrition, including *orthomolecular medicine,* is based on the belief that the genetic makeup of each individual is unique, with differing nutritional needs. Inadequate diets, environmental pollution, and stress rob food of its nutrients and are responsible for poorly assimilated vitamins, minerals, and amino acids, thereby causing illness. Orthomolecular refers to naturally occurring substances normally present in the body. Keeping these substances in proper balance and strength is imperative to good health.

Aromatherapy uses essential oils from plants to treat illnesses. The fragrance conveys the oils easily, and they are absorbed through body tissues. External and internal applications are used.

Bach flower remedies remove the emotional barriers to healing by helping to alleviate both psychological and physiological conditions that are detrimental to good health. Flower remedies work indirectly through the emotions to bring about physical healing through stimulation of the internal healing process.

Biofeedback teaches how to change and control the body's vital functions such as breathing, blood pressure, and heart rate through use of electronic devices. It is most commonly used for stress-related disorders.

Cell therapy is an injection of healthy cells from the organs, embryos, or fetuses of animals into the body. Used throughout Europe, it has not been approved for use in the United States. The main benefit of cell therapy is stimulation of the body processes, rejuvenating the patient.

Chelation therapy draws toxins and metabolic wastes from the bloodstream through intravenous injections of ethylene-diaminetetraacetic (EDTA). Treatments last about 3½ hours. They reduce the internal inflammation caused by free radicals that cause degenerative diseases such as arthritis and lupus, in addition to removing lead and other heavy metal toxins.

Colon therapy advocates a healthy colon for elimination of the buildup of toxins in the body. Water is introduced into the lower intestine to loosen impacted materials and detoxify the colon. Relief from a wide range of symptoms is possible, including headache and backache, bad breath, bloating, indigestion, skin problems, and constipation.

Detoxification therapy consists of a combination of alternative therapies aimed at ridding the body of the toxins and pollutants of modern times. The approach involves fasting, diets, colon therapy, vitamin therapy, chelation, and hyperthermia.

Enzyme therapy proposes that the ability to absorb nutrients from foods is dependent on enzymes. Remedying digestive disorders, then, is the first step toward restoration of good health. Plant-derived and pancreatic enzymes are used in this therapy to benefit both the digestive and the immune system. Enzyme therapy must be used in combination with proper diet to work effectively.

Fasting therapies give a powerful boost to the healing process. After 2 days of fasting on water or juice, the body's store of glucose is depleted, and fat is used for energy. Toxins stored in the fat cells are released and eliminated; the body's digestive system gets a rest, and the immune system is stimulated. There is increased oxygenation, and more white cells are activated.

Herbal medicine is derived from leaves, flowers, stems, seeds, roots, bark, fruits, or any part of a plant. Of the quarter to half million plants on earth, only 5,000 have been studied for their medicinal value. Herbs are generally used in teas, capsules, extracts, oils, and ointments. Information on herbal uses is well documented, and herbs are readily available to the general public.

Homeopathy is based on three principles: like cures like (the Law of Similars); the greater the dilution of a medicine, the more potent it is (the Law of Infinitesimal Dose); and, illness is individualistic and holistic. The Law of Similars was first promoted by Hippocrates around 400 BC and is based on the introduction of medicine that is similar to the disease, just as vaccines introduce live viruses in order to produce a reaction that protects (immunizes) the body. The Law of Infinitesimal Dose bases its validity from findings in the fields of quantum physics and energy medicine. Individual and holistic practice calls for a complete evaluation of the physical, mental, and emotional state of each patient, with the resulting remedies specific to that person alone.

Juice therapy consists of stimulating the immune system and causing detoxification through drinking raw fruit and vegetable juices. Juice therapies often consist of fasts lasting from 1 day to several weeks and are used for a variety of conditions, from prevention of illness to treatment of disease conditions ranging from colds to AIDS, depending on the medicinal qualities of the fruits and vegetables.

Macrobiotic therapy is built on a complicated system of food combining and consumption. Yin and yang energy foods are used during certain times of the day or season, and environmental conditions are factored in for optimum healing. A macrobiotic diet consists of whole cereal grains; fresh, locally grown vegetables; sea vegetables; beans; and fruit.

Naturopathy draws from many cultures and approaches to healing, including nutrition, acupuncture, herbal medicine, exercise, spinal manipulation, counseling, and homeopathy. It embraces six guiding principles: the healing power of nature, treating the cause rather than the effect, doing no harm, treating the whole person, the physician as teacher, and prevention as the best cure.

Oxygen therapy or *oxidating agent therapy* destroys pathogens through oxygenation of the blood or tissues or through oxidation, the reaction of splitting off electrons from any chemical molecule without harming healthy tissue and cells. Hyperbaric oxygen, hydrogen peroxide, and ozone therapies are all part of the oxygen therapy approach. They are administered under clinical supervision in a variety of ways—oral, vaginal, rectal, intravenous, inhalation, absorption, subcutaneous injection, and intraarterial.

MIND/SPIRIT HEALING

Art therapy uses interpretive techniques to assess a person's emotions and concerns through the symbolism in his or her drawings. Art therapy is also used for mental health rehabilitation.

Autogenic therapy, akin to hypnosis and meditation, consists of a systematic series of attention-focusing exercises designed for mind and body relaxation. These self-hypnotic techniques are taught so that they may be done several times a day without a therapist. Autogenic modification is directed toward a specific dysfunctional organ or body part in order to overcome certain chronic conditions such as allergies, bowel problems, weight gain or loss, or behavioral problems.

Charismatic Catholics, like most faith healers, believe miracles come from God or his saints. Divine healing and wisdom flows from the laying on of hands, speaking in tongues, and prayer vigils.

Christian Science is based on the teachings of Mary Baker Eddy, who published a book on fusing health and spirituality. Christian Science practitioners and nurses are licensed by the church, and treatment consists mainly of prayer. Unlike faith healers, they do not attribute cure to miracles from God; instead they tap into a divine principle that allows healing power to flow.

Color therapy relies on highly specialized equipment to project pure color for healing. Color is beamed on the body parts corresponding to the problem for a specified amount of time. Color is sometimes used in conjunction with application of healing oils.

Edgar Cayce remedies are based on the belief that in the mental and spiritual realms there is an antidote for every illness. Healing occurs when the vibrations from within are changed. Using drugless methods, the goals of treatment pursued are assimilation (utilization of food by the body), elimination (through intestines, kidneys, skin, and lungs), circulation, and relaxation.

Faith healing as practiced in the United States is primarily based on the Bible: laying on of hands, casting out of demons, releasing the patient's sins, praying, and anointing with oils. Several evangelical or pentecostal healers have achieved celebrity status through the media.

Guided imagery, or *visualization,* consists of a flow of thoughts that a person sees, feels, smells, hears, and tastes in his or her imagination. Appropriate images, first guided by a therapist, then practiced alone, can reduce stress, slow heart rate, lower blood pressure, stimulate the immune system, and influence numerous physiological activities of the body.

Humor therapy shows that laughter produces a positive physiological reaction to pain and disease through release of endorphins. Although it had been researched earlier, Norman Cousins popularized the effect of this healing in a book detailing his recovery from a diagnosed incurable disease.

Hypnotherapy induces a state of mind resulting in profound relaxation, conducive to bringing about beneficial psychological and physiological changes. Especially helpful for controlling pain, hypnotherapy also has been used as an aid and even a substitute for anesthesia.

Meditation balances a person's mind, body, and spirit through achievement of an altered level of relaxation and consciousness. In some Eastern practices, this is done through use of a mantra. Most practices emphasize deep breathing. Positive physiological and psychological changes that influence healing, manage pain, and reduce stress may occur in meditative states.

Music, sound therapy can slow breathing and blood pressure rates, alleviate pain, improve movement and balance, and influence brain wave frequencies. Sound is linked to the body through certain cranial nerves that carry impulses to the brain. Various sounds influence separate parts of the brain. Illness can occur when inner rhythms of the body are disturbed; sound therapy can restore health through its effect on the brain and, subsequently, physiological functions.

Past life, or regression, therapy developed from a growing awareness of ancient spiritual traditions and beliefs that illness in this life may be the result of unresolved conditions in past lives. Hypnosis or some form of altered consciousness is used to delve into memories from past times as therapist and client/patient work together to bring about healing and understanding.

Psychic healing draws on help from powers or beings from another realm. Like faith healers, psychics may practice through the laying on of hands, but they often just touch the person's aura or magnetic field. Psychics support or catalyze the subject's own healing energy and mechanisms.

Psychotherapy uses a variety of techniques to achieve a healing from within the person. Mind-body connections are most important and are often combined with imagery, relaxation techniques, and hypnotherapy.

CROSS-CULTURAL HEALING

Acupuncture and *acupressure* originated in China more than 5,000 years ago and are based on the belief that good health results from that balanced flow of energy called *chi* (or *qi*). Energy circulates in the body through 12 meridians, each of which is linked to an organ. When needles are inserted (or pressure is used) on the acupuncture points, this helps to restore the flow or energy, thereby alleviating pain and enhancing the immune system.

Ayurvedic medicine originated in India 5,000 years ago and places equal emphasis on body, mind, and spirit to restore harmony to the individual. Identification of a person's constitution through his or her metabolic body type (*dosha*) is essential to treatment. Special attention is paid to the pulse, tongue, eyes, and nails.

Chi gong, or qigong, is an ancient Chinese exercise system that stimulates and balances the flow of *chi* (vital life energy). *Chi* is directed through exercises or through touch by a *chi qong* master to the site of an injury and facilitates the signals to the brain stem. As a result of increased blood and lymph flow, a greater supply of nutrients is delivered to the injured area, regenerating the cells and healing the injury.

Curanderismo is folk medicine, first practiced in Central and South America. Combining herbal medicines with religion, *curanderos* act as specialists in medical information and healing for Hispanic cultures in the United States.

Folk medicine in the United States originally combined the healing techniques of European colonists with those of Native Americans. Still evident today in Appalachia and dispersed throughout the United States, folk medicine is based on a sense that everyone should be his or her own doctor. Healing herbs are made into remedies dispensed by lay practitioners. A major work on folk healing was self-published by Jethro Kloss (1939) and continues to be a popular book.

Jin shin jyutsu came from Japan and treats patients by holding a combination of healing points along the *qi* flow for 1 to 5 minutes. Treatments are performed in a meditative state to promote mind and body balance.

Moxibustion therapy is a Chinese healing technique that uses *moxa* (cigarlike mugwort herbs) sticks lit at one end and held close to acupressure points corresponding to the painful areas. This is continued until the skin turns pink and feels very hot but is not burned. In acupuncture the needles are lit by burning mugwort.

Native American medicine men/women conduct elaborate healing ceremonies passed down through generations using the oral tradition. Ceremonies are tailored to the individual's need for balance in nature and sometimes call for herbal medicines, hallucinogenic drugs, prayers, medicine wheels, and sweat lodges to evoke healing spirits and/or enter states of altered consciousness to cleanse and heal both body and mind.

Reiki massage originated in Japan; *reiki* means universal life force energy. The therapist is a conduit for healing coming from the universe, with the energy entering through the therapist's head and exiting through the hands. Stones such as crystals and quartz are believed to have special qualities and are sometimes placed on the client.

Shamanism is practiced in native cultures around the globe. Believing that all healing comes from the spiritual dimension, shamans enter altered states of consciousness. Different cultures imprint their own practices, but underlying most is a respect for nature and a sense of our place *in* nature, not over it. Healing occurs when one is in balance and harmony with nature.

Shiatsu, similar to reflexology, is a Japanese technique that applies finger pressure for 3 to 10 seconds in a sequence of specific points to activate the energy along the body's meridians.

Tai chi integrates aspects of the Chinese Tao and Buddhism into a gentle system of exercise emphasizing strength and flexibility. It is derived from the martial arts and, using smooth, nonaerobic movements, tai chi contains rather than expends energy.

Traditional Chinese medicine is a complex system that is difficult to describe adequately in a few sentences. Briefly, it uses medicinal herbs, diet, exercise, massage, and acupuncture and focuses largely on prevention. Pathways called meridians allow energy (*chi*) to flow freely in a healthy person. Blockages in these pathways interrupt *chi* and result in disease in a particular organ. The diseased organ can be accessed through applying pressure on the meridian, either manually or with needles. This, in combination with diet, medicinal herbs, and exercise, restores balance and health.

Voodoo originated in Africa, coming to the Caribbean through slave ships. *Vou do* priests and priestesses employ a variety of healing mechanisms, including medicinal herbs, animal parts, trances, healing touch, spells, dancing, singing, and prayer to dispel spirit-caused illness.

Witch doctors derive from the shaman tradition and use cures, spells, and hexes to remove disease caused by evil spirits. These are often supplemented with herbal medicine.

Yoga techniques consist of using stretching postures (hatha-yoga), breathing (*kundalini* yoga), and meditations to relieve stress and restore health and vitality. Physiological changes are experienced in blood rate and heartbeat reductions, enhanced metabolic and respiratory functions, and pain alleviation.

Index

Numbers followed by *t* refer to tables; numbers followed by *f* refer to figures.

S *Springer Publishing Company*

Wellness Practitioner
Concepts, Theory, Research, Strategies, and Programs, 2nd Edition

Carolyn Chambers Clark, EdD, ARNP

Now in a second edition, this is a comprehensive resource on health maintenance, disease prevention, and alternative health practices. The author explores conceptual bases and practical techniques for a wide range of programs, activities, and therapies that promote wellness. Topics include relaxation and stress management, nutrition, exercise, herbal remedies, massage, imagery, affirmations, reflexology, aromatherapy, natural healing, and self care measures for conditions ranging from hay fever to multiple sclerosis.

Environmental influences and community wellness are each addressed in a separate chapter. Learning exercises are included with each chapter to facilitate integration of the material. A useful resource for nurses, physicians, and other health professionals — both traditional and alternative.

Partial Contents
- Introduction to Wellness Theory
- Beginning to Move Toward Wellness
- Positive Relationship Building
- Stress Management
- Nutritional Wellness
- Exercise and Movement
- Self-Care, Touch, and Wellness

1996   354pp   0-8261-5151-5   hardcover

536 Broadway, New York, NY 10012-3955 • (212) 431-4370 • Fax (212) 941-7842

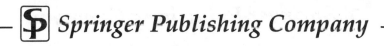

Springer Publishing Company

Complementary / Alternative Therapies in Nursing, 3rd Edition

Mariah Snyder, PhD, RN, FAAN
Ruth Lindquist, PhD, RN

This book offers a systematic approach to a wide range of complementary/alternative therapies that can be used by nurses independently. Each of the chapters describes a different therapy and follows a standard format: definition, review of current research, description of uses and techniques, precautions, and a list of questions for further research.

Many of these therapies such as massage and application of heat and cold have traditionally been part of nursing practice, while others such as imagery, meditation, and biofeedback are interventions that nurses can use to enrich their practice. Students and clinicians in all specialty areas of nursing will find this a straightforward and practical resource.

Contents: Progressive Muscle Relaxation, *M. Snyder* • Breathing, *J. Wang and M. Snyder* • Exercise, *D. Treat-Jacobson and D.L. Mark* • Tai Chi/Movement Therapy, *K. Shaller* • Therapeutic Touch, *E. Egan* • Massage, *M. Snyder and W. Cheng* • Biofeedback, *M. Good* • Application of Heat and Cold, *S. Ridgeway, D. Brauer, J. Corso, J. Daniels, and M. Steffes* • Imagery, *J. Post-White* • Meditation, *M.J. Kreitzer* • Aromatherapy, *K. James* • Purposeful Touch, *M. Snyder and Y. Nojima* • Presence, *S. Moch and C. Schaefer* • Active Listening, *M. Ryden* • Positioning, *M.F. Tracy* • Sensation Information, *J. Ruiz-Bueno* • Journal Writing, *M. Snyder* • Reminiscence, *M. Snyder* • Story Telling, *P. Dicke* • Validation Therapy, *L. Taft* • Music Therapy, *L. Chlan* • Prayer, *M. Gustafon* • Humor, *K. Smith* • Pet Therapy, *K. James* • Contracting, *R. Lindquist* • Groups, *M. Kaas and M.F. Richie* • Family Support, *M. Mirr* • Advocacy, *M. Nelson*

1998   376pp (est)   0-8261-1169-6   hardcover

536 Broadway, New York, NY 10012-3955 • (212) 431-4370 • Fax (212) 941-7842

⑤ *Springer Publishing Company*

Nutrition Policy in Public Health
Felix Bronner, PhD, Editor

This is the first book to deal comprehensively with nutrition policy in the public health of the United States. It combines theoretical and practical approaches to integrating nutrition concepts into public health planning with research and intervention strategies.

The book also summarizes international policies, calling attention to what has and hasn't worked, and focuses on what nutritionists can do and the knowledge they need to do it. The many dimensions of the relationship between nutrition and disease (an obvious but complex and controversial topic) and what counsel nutritionists can provide a concerned public are covered in detail. The book stresses the complex interaction among nutrients, lifestyles, genetic makeup, and health.

Contents:

General Aspects of Nutrition Policy. Nutrition Policy in Public Health: Rationale and Approaches • Behavior and Food Intake: What Constitutes Effective Policy • Food-Borne Health Risks: Food Additives, Pesticides and Microbes • Legal Aspects of Food Protection • Food: Production, Processing, Distribution, and Consumption

Nutrition-Related Conditions and Diseases—Policies and Approaches. Intervention Strategies for Undernutrition • The Obesity Epidemic: Nutrition Policy and Public Health Imperatives • Coronary Heart Disease and Public Health Nutrition • Nutrition in the Etiology, Prevention, Control and Treatment of Cancer • Osteoporosis • Dental Caries Prevention • Selected Disease Entities: AIDS, Alcoholism, Diabetes Mellitus, Lead and Lead Poisoning, Neural Tube Defects, Nutritional Anemias

Nutrition Policies and Approaches Targeted at Populations at Risk. Pregnant Mothers and Their Young Children: The WIC Program • Issues in Development of a Nutrition Policy for Preschool and School-Aged Children • Nutrition Policy for the Elderly

Nutrition Policy Perspective. Opportunities and Challenges of New Nutrition Environments: International Experiences and Implications for U.S. Policymaking

1997   345pp   0-8261-9660-8   hardcover

536 Broadway, New York, NY 10012-3955 • (212) 431-4370 • Fax (212) 941-7842